Spirituality

The Heart
of
Nursing

Edited by Professor Susan Ronaldson

Foreword by Professor Mary Bailey

AUSMED PUBLICATIONS
MELBOURNE

Australasian Health Education Systems Pty Ltd
(ACN 005 611 727)
trading as
Ausmed Publications
275 Mount Alexander Road
Ascot Vale, Victoria 3032, Australia

First published August 1997
Reprinted 2000

Further copies of this book and of all other Ausmed publications are available from
the Distribution Manager, Ausmed Publications, PO Box 4086, Melbourne
University, Victoria 3052, Australia.
Telephone: +61 3 9375 7311.
Fax: +61 3 9375 7299.
E-mail ausmed@ausmed.com.au

National Library of Australia Cataloguing-in-Publication data:
Spirituality: the heart of nursing
Includes bibliographical references and index

ISBN 0 646 32259 1.
1. Nursing - Religious aspects. 2. Nursing - Psychological aspects. 3. Nursing -
Philosophy. I. Ronaldson, Susan, 1953- .
610.7301

Edited by Robyn Whiteley, The WC Company Pty Ltd
Cover, design and typesetting by Colorperception Pty Ltd

Text set in 11/15pt Sabon

Printed in Australia by Australian Print Group

ʃpirituality

The Heart
of
Nursing

To nurses who value

their role as a spiritual carer

The title of this book was suggested by the original title of
Rosemary Lancaster's chapter, which was
'Spirituality: the heart of caring'. We thank her for allowing
us to adapt her title.

FOREWORD

Modern medicine has brought the marvels of cure to infections and has certainly been responsible for linking technology and cure to life-threatening conditions. At the same time technology's very success has been its major failure. Scientific medicine finds it difficult to answer important questions put forward by our patients — namely questions of the *meaning* of illness, disability and death. Patients are left alone to cope as scientifically based 20th century medicine continues to search for the 'ultimate machine', pharmaceutical agent or surgery to cure patient ills.

To adequately *care* for patients, the nursing profession is viewing Care as the 'ability to journey with patients and to answer important questions related to nursing' — these are questions involving the spiritual domain.

Today there is a growing questioning of an all-encompassing reliance on science as it is linked to cure and healing.

Healing is dependent on 'seeing wholes' — not parts or systems only of a human being. Healing is dependent not only on focusing on a diseased organ but on listening to how that disease impacts on a patient's life and family. Healing might include a variety of possible treatments and takes into account much more than the scientific method allows for consideration. Healing views man as body, mind and spirit. Mind and spirit, and especially spirit, are given little attention as science seeks only what can be objectified, and experimentally proven.

In the 1990s nurses continue to work harder and longer in a rationalised system of Care — the results of a 'market' or business approach to care. Yet many surveys report these are not happy times and nurses are not finding fulfilment in the work environment (*American Journal of Nursing*, November 1996). In fact many recent studies within the United States present data that nurses will exit the nursing profession in increasing numbers as they seek fulfilment, value and meaning elsewhere. And patients too are not satisfied with Health Care today.

What could be the cause of this dilemma? Could this also happen in Australia? The need to recognise the spiritual side of Care will bring some answers to these questions and concerns.

In this fine book on Spirituality and Nursing we experience the bringing together of varied and seasoned clinicians and their reflection of the human predicament. These reflections will inspire and lead the way as nurse colleagues face the practice issues of the millennium.

Part of the way we learn about 'the spiritual domain' is by listening to others' stories. This fine book continues the process of learning from the stories of nurses — nurses who are discovering the joy of entering, with patients and families, the spiritual dimension of Care.

So let us begin . . .

Mary Pfiester Bailey, PhD, RN
Professor of Nursing and International Health
Madonna University
Livonia, Michigan
USA

Contents

INTRODUCTION
Nurses as spiritual carers

Sue Ronaldson

Recently at a public forum I was surprised to hear the question asked: *Is it really the nurse's role to provide spiritual care?* Why was I surprised? Because to me, nurses are spiritual carers. For me, the question represents a limited view of both nursing and spirituality. If spiritual care is not provided by nurses, both the nurse and the person in need of such care are impoverished. Nurses provide spiritual care often as a subtext to their caring role. It is now time to recognise, articulate and claim this important element of nursing. While spiritual beliefs are generally considered to be a private concern, the need for spiritual caring is often foremost for individuals when challenges to health occur. The meaning of one's life and purpose, sense of hope, and belief in oneself and a power beyond self, are confronted and questioned. Nurses have a presence in these times of significant stress and turmoil. They are there to listen, to reflect, to clarify and, importantly, to foster hope.

Nurses, as health professionals, work in the health industry — a service industry. Here I am reminded of a single event which I now recognise as a spiritual one — an awakening which emerges periodically in my work and which holds great meaning for me. This spiritual awakening occurred as I was drying the feet of an elderly man residing in a large aged care facility in north-east Victoria. I was working as an educator of student nurses. For a brief moment in time I was struck by the translucency and radiance of the thin, pale, aged skin on this man's feet. This caring act represented to me the service role of nursing. I then understood at a very deep level that I was both immensely privileged and humbled to possess the skills to perform such a relatively simple, yet enormously important, act of caring. I was performing a most valuable

1

human task — being at one with the needs of this undemanding and vulnerable elderly man. Much later I was to recognise this was an experience of 'vernacular spirituality', an appreciation of the sacred in the ordinary (Sexson, 1982, in Moore, 1994:215). It was the beginnings of my identity as a gerontic nurse and the confirmation of the meaning of nursing in my life.

Nurses, in their many and varied roles, are in a pivotal position to provide spiritual caring. An understanding of the spiritual self will carve a niche in nurses' abilities to provide truly holistic care. *Spirituality: The Heart of Nursing* describes nurses as spiritual carers and unravels the place of spirituality in nursing. It not only invites nurses to explore spiritual caring, it challenges them to identify the meaning of spirituality in both their personal and professional lives.

Interest in the concept of spirituality has increased markedly over the past decade and is reflected in both general and health care literature. Much discussion occurs in *Spirituality: The Heart of Nursing* in relation to the importance of identifying spirituality and religion as separate yet related concepts. Authors discuss the place for spiritual assessment and the need for nurses to provide spiritual care. Some discuss the history of spiritual care in relation to people's health needs while others explore concepts relevant to spirituality in nursing, such as nurses as wounded healers, power and powerlessness, and the relatedness of spiritual philosophies to nursing. Parts of this book explore the meaning of spirituality for people when they are challenged by illness or impending death. There are writings on the place of spiritual care for specific individuals: elderly people, older people with dementia, and those in need of palliative care, and mental health nursing. The chapter titles chosen by each of the authors are descriptive of their content

Major concepts which weave through this book are the need for individuals to maintain hope and to preserve self-determination.

Collectively the authors stress the need for nurses' expansion of their present concepts of spirituality and of nursing, and urge them to address each individual's spiritual self.

Through the reading of *Spirituality: The Heart of Nursing* I hope that you also will become aware of the apposition of the practice of nursing with the meanings of spirituality and nursing for you, and for those for whom you care. 'Spirituality is seeded, germinates, sprouts and blossoms in the mundane. It is found and nurtured in the smallest of daily activities . . . the spirituality that feeds the soul and ultimately heals our psychological wounds may be found in those sacred objects that dress themselves in the accoutrements of the ordinary' (Moore, 1994:219).

Spirituality and nursing are historically and inextricably interwoven. 'The soul needs spirit, but our spirituality also needs soul — deep intelligence, a sensitivity to the symbolic and metaphoric life, genuine community, and attachment to the world' (Moore, 1994:229). Nursing's philosophy of care and its founding beliefs are commensurate with these concepts. As the title eloquently suggests, Spirituality is at the Heart of Nursing. Our quest is to reimagine both spirituality and nursing in our everyday and professional lives.

REFERENCE

Moore T (1994): *Care of the Soul, A Guide for Cultivating Depth and Sacredness in Everyday* . New York: Harper Perennial.

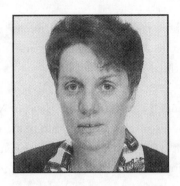

ANNE J. FRY
RN, BA (Macq), MLitt (UNE), MRCNA, MRANZCMHN

Anne Fry is conjointly appointed as a Senior Lecturer in Mental Health Nursing by the Faculty of Nursing and Health Studies at the University of Western Sydney — Nepean and the Blacktown City Mental Health Service, both in New South Wales, Australia.

Anne has a clinical nursing background in community mental health nursing in inner Sydney and general nursing in Canberra. As a nurse academic, Anne has been in higher education for ten years and has worked at three universities. Her current interests include doctoral studies on the topic of 'Spirituality and mental health nursing', suicide prevention, cross-cultural mental health and mental health nursing. Her professional priorities include promoting nursing through research in partnership with nurse practitioners.

Chapter 1

SPIRITUALITY:
CONNECTEDNESS THROUGH BEING
AND DOING

In contrast with other disciplines in health care, nursing has long been concerned with the religious and spiritual dimension of personhood. Spirituality is a part of the 'ontological foundation of nursing; it is regarded as a basic characteristic of humanness important in human health and well being' (Reed, 1992:350). However, its recognition, explication of meaning, the way it is experienced and its impact on the lives and work of nurses and patients, have not been well addressed in the nursing literature. The commitment of the nursing profession to the notion of spirituality and its implications for practice has also been inconsistent and remains controversial.

This chapter addresses three aspects of spirituality. The concept of spirituality and its historical place in nursing are outlined. Reasons for the neglect of spirituality in nursing theory, education and practice are reviewed. Finally, a reflection on spirituality and work highlights a spiritual orientation to mental health nursing practice.

HISTORY, SPIRITUALITY AND NURSING

The root meanings of spiritual terms are, in Hebrew, *rauch* (Smith, 1988) and *ruah* (Dickinson, 1975); in Greek, *psyche* (Smith, 1988) and *pneuma* (Dickinson, 1975); and, from the Latin, *spiritus* (Smith, 1988; Dickinson, 1975). These all borrow metaphorically the phenomenon of moving air, breath and wind (Smith, 1988), and the breath of life (Dickinson, 1975). Spirit refers to the animating life force of human beings and may be defined and understood in diverse ways according to different religious, cultural and philosophical traditions.

Reed (1992) conceptualised spirituality as a propensity to make meaning through a sense of relatedness/connectedness to dimensions that transcend the self in a way that empowers and does not devalue the individual. This relatedness may be experienced via three dimensions: intrapersonally — by having purpose, satisfaction and values; interpersonally — through giving and receiving in relationships; and transpersonally — by a link with a higher being (Reed, 1992:350).

The attributes of spirituality include: innateness (Chandler, Holden and Kolander, 1992); a capacity for inner knowing and a source of strength (Burkhardt, 1994); subjective experience of the sacred (Vaughan, 1995); self-transcendence toward a capacity for greater love and knowledge (Chandler, Holden and Kolander, 1992); a 'unity or wholeness permeating all of one's life' (Burkhardt, 1994:15); and provision of meaning of one's existence that lies at the core of one's being (MacKinlay, 1996).

The nature of people as spiritual beings and the connection of spirituality with healing are two reasons which explain the importance of the spiritual in nursing. Spirituality is a profound and central aspect of the existence of many people. As nursing is concerned with the care of the whole person, it is also concerned with spiritual life (as relevant to individual patients). Both spirituality and nursing are enmeshed in the life experience of people.

Secondly, spirituality, has an important impact on the power of recovery and the ability to cope with and adjust to varying states of health and illness (Oldnall, 1995; Reed, 1992; Ross, 1994).

The individual's perception of the meaning, purpose and fulfilment of life have [*sic*] the ability to create a sense of hopelessness/helplessness that can ultimately exert a dramatic influence over the individual, resulting in physical and mental illness, which may ultimately determine the individual's quality of life (Oldnall, 1995:417).

The nursing profession recognises spirituality in the accepted diagnostic classification system, the North American Nursing Diagnoses Association (NANDA) (Kim, McFarland and McLane, 1987). The nursing diagnosis of 'spiritual distress' is defined as a 'disruption in the life principle which pervades a person's entire being and which integrates and transcends one's biological and psychological nature' (Kim, McFarland and McLane, 1987:55).

Historically, the origins of the spiritual perspective of nursing evolved from the role of medieval Christian religious orders who cared for the sick (Hall and Lanig, 1993) as a 'good work' necessary for salvation. As such, this tradition incorporated certain values about the nature of humans as spiritual beings. Consistent with this tradition Florence Nightingale, who developed a deep spirituality originating during her formative years in the Anglican Christian tradition, laid the foundations of modern nursing, incorporating her philosophy of spirituality into nursing theory and practice (Macrae, 1995). Nightingale believed that spirituality is intrinsic to human nature and is our deepest and most potent resource for healing (Macrae, 1995).

Despite this early awareness of the spiritual dimension in nursing, spirituality was ignored and forgotten in mainstream secular nursing practice, education and inquiry for a century or more, in contrast with other nursing foci. Spirituality is viewed as one of the dimensions of personhood but the notion has received relatively little attention. Spirituality was rendered, by neglect, the illegitimate and somewhat embarrassing offspring of a religious past no longer relevant to the modern, scientific world of biomedical science.

Remarkably, however, in the latter twentieth century, there is a resurgence of interest in spirituality in nursing and other health disciplines. Recent nursing literature abounds with references to spirituality in diverse practice and theoretical contexts. As Dombeck (1995) states, a body of knowledge in nursing theory, practice and research has emerged, emphasising the distinct and important contribution of the nursing profession to the spiritual care of persons. Yet the debate is characterised by conceptual and semantic confusion, with such terms as spirituality and religion being used interchangeably, whereas both are heterogenous, multidimensional constructs.

The earlier lack of nursing literature and research in the area (Ross, 1994) resulted in the topic not being seen, in the past, as a worthwhile endeavour for nurse scholars but the situation is rapidly reversing. There is a notable absence of reference to spirituality in nursing theories and models (Oldnall, 1995) although this trend is changing. In the 1970s Betty Neuman's systems theory omitted the concept of spirituality, but in the late 1980s it was included in a revised version of the theory (Meleis, 1991). Other nursing theorists, such as Parse (Parse, 1987) and Watson (Meleis, 1991), have a major focus on spirituality. Certainly spirituality has long been implicitly acknowledged in the conceptual framework of nursing which espouses the holistic approach to care, but little emphasis was placed on this dimension so fundamental to many consumers of nursing services. In education programs, spirituality is often superficially addressed and subsumed under psychological care (Narayanasamy, 1993).

ACCOUNTING FOR THE LOW PRIORITY OF THE SPIRITUAL IN NURSING EDUCATION AND PRACTICE

The neglect of spirituality in education and practice settings may be accounted for by many factors. Conceptual and semantic difficulties, reluctance to explore the private and personal, gender differences, fear, characteristics of certain practice settings, cultural value biases, historical derivatives, professional role delineations and patient difficulties in communicating inhibit the exploration of spirituality in nursing theory and practice in Australia.

The conceptual confusion between religion and spirituality, the lack of clarity in definition, conceptual overlap and vague terminology have not encouraged scholars in nursing to explore spirituality. The word spiritual is being used as an umbrella term that includes 'awareness of personal transcendence, personal relationships, and interpersonal communications as well as the traditional beliefs and practices' (Emblem and Halstead, 1993:175). Furthermore, spiritual terminology may have been avoided for fear of being unscientific.

According to Oldnall (1995) the concept of spirituality is nebulous and not easily quantified. Consequently, he argues, it does not lend itself to scientific exploration and lacks credibility as a worthy subject in nursing's efforts to establish itself as a scientific discipline. The contextualisation of spirituality within the positivistic/scientific paradigm in Oldnall's (1995) argument betrays a bias that any truth/knowledge obtained from other ways of knowing, such as those represented in qualitative methodologies, are less valuable. Subjective paths to knowing have been equated with women's ways of knowing (Belenky et al., 1986, as cited in Streubert and Carpenter, 1995) which, according to feminist ideologies, are devalued by patriarchal purveyors of 'truth' throughout history. Nevertheless, this attitude may well prevail and in part explain the neglect of the topic. Basically, spirituality is not a well-understood phenomenon despite its fascination for scholars and ordinary people for millennia.

The personal nature of spirituality may also be a factor in academics' failure to comprehend the impact of spirituality on the individual and include it in educational programs for nurses (Harrington, 1995; Oldnall, 1995). Questions about spiritual experience can be difficult and threatening (Stiles, 1994). The implication is that issues that have the potential to cause embarrassment have historically been ignored by the profession as a defence against the anxiety-arousing potential of the topic. This anxiety may be related to association of spirituality with death and dying (Harrington, 1995). In holistic care, spirituality has been likened to sexuality — conveniently brushed over because it is regarded as too intimate and private for the public sphere (Oldnall, 1995). However, a study by Harrington (1995) noted that intimacy regarding biological functioning, such as elimination, menstruation and sexual functioning, was allowable because these fall into the accepted biomedical model for care.

In contrast, fears of intrusion into the client's privacy regarding the spiritual domain inhibited nurses from interacting with clients about spirituality (Harrington, 1995). Such sensitivities are obviously appropriate for a great deal of the time in nursing, but recognition of spiritual needs may also be crucial at certain occasions, such as life transitions and crises. The lack of guidelines for practice in the area of spirituality has led to the recommendation that educators and supervisors should not push nurses into spiritual intervention 'until they demonstrate readiness' (Hall and Lanig, 1993:739). The notion of readiness presupposes that nurses want to develop skills in the area of intervention and that it is appropriate to do so. However, discretion must determine the efficacy and wisdom of how this is to be done and when, if at all.

Time is also a pertinent factor which is governed by the nature of the clinical area. Certain clinical settings, such as hospices and palliative care settings, are more oriented to spiritual care. In contrast, 'cure-oriented care settings where the focus tends to be on diseases rather than on people' (Harrington, 1995:13) were perceived by nurses as too difficult for the provision of spiritual care because of lack of time. The rapid turnover of patients and the system of reimbursement based on casemix/diagnoses-related groups (Harrington, 1995) exacerbates the time pressure. The demands of rapid care services in busy acute care areas must not be underestimated as a factor that militates against the development of interpersonal communication between nurse and patient and, correspondingly, against the addressing of spiritual issues. Space is another crucial issue when the environment lacks quiet and privacy (Ross, 1994). Communication difficulties with the patient, notably deafness and dementia, have also been identified as interfering with giving spiritual care (Ross, 1994).

Gender differences are apparent in the research pertaining to spirituality. In a study by Emblem and Halstead (1993), male patients in the clinical setting were reluctant to discuss spirituality and male nurses reported reservations about discussing personal issues such as spirituality. There are substantially more female participants than males in numerous data-based nursing studies on spirituality. This phenomenon may be explained by cultural biases about masculinity which represent manliness and strength as antithetical to things spiritual.

Secularism is cited as a salient feature of Australian culture by Patience (1991:31) who describes Australian culture as 'hard' and 'impervious to some of the most civilised values that humankind has invented'. Religious commitment is equated with feminine nostalgia, which has no place in the public arena (Patience, 1991). Hostility and apathy remain the dominant approaches to religion in the hard culture (Patience, 1991).

From a historical perspective, according to Cleasby (1996:11), the origins of Australia as a penal colony influenced the 'pace and purpose of religion among descendants and future settlers' and, by extrapolation, negative or indifferent attitudes toward things spiritual. Cleasby (1996) argues that the cultural derivatives of the harsh penal settlement led to a view of religion that was negative, God-rejecting and authority-resenting. Christianity was seen as irrelevant in the early colony and the rich metaphysical speculation of various Aboriginal religions was ignored (Patience, 1991).

As nursing occurs in the cultural context of the Western world we incorporate the values of that world, which are oriented to the rationalistic, external world of the individual. In this value system, external world things and instrumental mastery are valued above the inner experience of meanings and affects (Williams, 1970). Spirituality is antithetical to this value orientation. In contrast, people in many other cultures have been aware of themselves as having spirit as well as body and as being influenced by spiritual energies and spiritual presences (Evans, 1993).

Finally, spiritual care may be seen as the realm of the chaplains or other pastoral workers (Narayanasamy, 1993; Cleasby, 1996) and outside the role of nurses. Nurses refer patients to chaplains when spiritual needs are recognised (Emblem and Halstead, 1993; Ross, 1994) partly because of lack of confidence in their ability to provide spiritual care (Harrington, 1995; Ross, 1994).

SPIRITUALITY AND WORK

Work is spirituality and spirituality is work. Although this saying is tautological and quizzical, it suggests that our working life is vitally connected to the spiritual. It also suggests that development of spirituality is an active not a passive process. Nursing as work (and mental health nursing specifically) is examined in the following section for insights about the nexus between spirituality and nursing. 'Being with' and 'doing with' our clients establishes a connectedness with them which is integral to healing and spirituality.

Recognition of nursing work as a spiritual experience is attributed to Florence Nightingale by Macrae (1995) and more recently by Barker (1996). Work, according to Nightingale, is performed not for personal gain but for itself. Macrae (1995) likens Nightingale's view of work to that of karma yoga from Hindu philosophy. As such, nursing the sick can be transformed into a spiritual discipline based on confidence that 'nature alone cures'. Nursing is about facilitating healing and focuses on the process of providing quality care in partnership with persons/patients and their families.

Nightingale held that finding work for which one is suited and performing it in simplicity and singleness of heart was the highest form of prayer. 'Work your true work, she wrote, and you will find God within you' (Macrae, 1995:10). A spiritual approach to life focuses on the other, and relegates into second place the needs of the ego for recognition and success. In contrast, the emphasis in our work environments these days is on outcome orientation, quantification and dissemination of success. Competition, power, status and achievement are only antithetical to spirituality when the other (or the self) is diminished in the process.

The essence of spirituality and its relationship with work is captured in a story narrated by Thomas Merton, a modern-day mystic.

A Russian 'Staretz' (holy monk) was criticised for spending time attentively advising an old peasant woman about the care of her turkeys (instead of going about the serious and important business of spiritual counselling). In reply he said 'not at all . . . her whole life is in those turkeys' (Merton, 1960:16).

In this sense, from the tradition of the Christian mystics, spirituality relates to the whole person in the concrete circumstances of his/her life (Merton, 1960:16) however simple or awesomely creative they may be. The only way we can know ourselves and others is within the context of our concrete personal world — our lived experience. For most of us the world of work is a major component of our life and for nurses it demands an intimate connection with human beings in various states of health and illness. The more we become present to ourselves, the more we get in touch with our spirituality. Human beings are entities of wholeness, and spirituality has the potential for permeation of a person's entire life.

As mental health nurses, we can identify with both the turkey woman and the holy man. We all have our own 'turkeys' or forms of work which demand time and commitment. The issue is not type or superiority of turkey but rather that work is, by definition, a productive or operative process. To be spiritual or connected to a 'higher reality' consists of doing what we should be doing when we should be doing it. For a large part of our lives this involves work, paid or unpaid. Work is important for many reasons, not the least of which is that our work, to an extent, defines us and contributes to our identity.

Mental health nurses have therapeutic relationships with disturbed clients. These are healing relationships and at times the healing extends to spiritual healing. Like the 'holy monk', in order to connect with clients and promote healing, including spiritual healing, we talk to clients about the concrete realities of their lives. Talking 'with' requires some of the specialist skills of our role including active listening, attentiveness, genuineness and comprehending the experience of psychotic symptoms such as hallucinations and delusions on the client's daily life. The nurse's personal spiritual interests are rarely made explicit because the skilled nurse is focused on the other, alert and responsive to cues that signal whatever is meaningful in the client's life. This affirming interaction is the medium for connecting with clients in deep dialogue and this is where spiritual healing can take place. The work is pure being with clients.

In another sense, spirituality is manifested by 'doing' work. Doing is a theme identified in a study of Appalachian women by Burkhardt (1994) who described it as the active component of spirituality which may involve work such as taking care of family, elderly parents or friends. The key element of work as spirituality was seen by these women in relation to others and described as connectedness. Mental health nursing actively connects with clients by sharing experiences with them such as planning a program of care and implementing it, referring to other facilities, having a cup of tea and discussing things, providing information, administering medication, participating in leisure activities in in-patient units.

At another level, work which engenders connectedness may involve more than human interrelationships and the nurse may promote the client's connectedness with nature and the earth, as in gardening and caring for the environment or by opening aesthetic windows for them such as the sheer appreciation of the beauty of nature, art and music. A sense of connectedness experienced through activity is linked to a desire for preservation and protectiveness. It follows that, where spirituality is weak, destructiveness and insidious neglect of the planet can lead to devastation.

The spirituality of nurses and their work has a delicate balance. A high level of spirituality is realised not by the amount of work we accomplish but rather the purity of heart with which we seek and love the sacred/higher reality, however we define it. The development of spirituality is thus described as a maturation process which requires quality time for quiet reflection. Working to extremes retards spiritual development because quality time and quiet reflection tend to be undervalued and neglected. Work is not a substitute for spiritual development, even if we are particularly good at it. The notion of doing one's duty in productive work should not become excessive 'busyness' to the exclusion of balance in life. Elisabeth Kübler-Ross (cited in Vaughan, 1995, p. 772), who spent decades caring for the dying and writing about her experiences, said that most people on their deathbed regretted not having taken more time for relationship in life. No-one ever regretted spending too little time at the office, but rather, too little time in relationship development, that is, in their connections with others.

Kübler-Ross (1975: xi) observed that:

To rejoice at the opportunity of experiencing each new day is to prepare for one's ultimate acceptance of death. For it is those who have not really lived — who have left issues unsettled, dreams unfulfilled, hopes shattered, and who have let the real things in life (loving and being loved by others, contributing in a positive way to other people's happiness and welfare, finding out what things are really you) pass them by — who are most reluctant to die.

To really live one's life, therefore, is to achieve satisfaction in the balance of leisure, stillness, relationship development and work. Spirituality is enhanced by the harmony of balance.

Thomas Merton (1960:85) states that 'the highest spiritual good is an action which is so perfect that it is absolutely free of all labour, and is therefore at the same time perfect action and perfect rest. And this is the contemplation of God.' Such advanced meditation is a process that not many of us achieve in our generally pressured lives. As most of us are not mystics, we tend to cope day to day the best we can, generally striving for excellence in our practice. Work is a necessary part of human existence and at the end of the day cannot be avoided. Whatever the heights of spiritual enlightenment attained, one must live in the world grounded in the reality of the basic needs of the body and social obligation. The spiritual heights reached do not preclude living in the real world with real obligations and routine tasks. According to Vaughan (1995) after reaching enlightenment in the Buddhist tradition, one must first return to the world and assist others along the way. This requires 'forgiving the past, accepting one's spiritual roots and sharing what has been discovered' (Vaughan, 1995:22). Secondly, one must manage the basic chores of life. As they say in Zen, 'before enlightenment, chop wood and carry water. After enlightenment, chop wood and carry water' (Vaughan, 1995:22).

REFERENCES

Barker PJ (1996): The logic of experience: developing appropriate care through effective collaboration. *Australian and New Zealand Journal of Mental Health Nursing* 5: 3-12.

Burkhardt MA (1994): Becoming and connecting: elements of spirituality for women. *Holistic Nursing Practice* 8 4: 12-21.

Chandler CK, Holden JM, Kolander CA (1992): Counselling for spiritual wellness: theory and practice. *Journal of Counselling and Development* Nov.–Dec. 71: 169-175.

Cleasby P (1996): Spirituality care in nursing — a forgotten path. *Spirituality in Nursing Practice*. Papers from a conference held on 27 March 1996 at The Swiss Grand Hotel, Bondi, Australia. Melbourne: Ausmed Publications.

Dickinson C (1975): The search for spiritual meaning. *American Journal of Nursing* 75 10: 1789-1793.

Dombeck MT (1995): Dream telling: a means of spiritual awareness. *Holistic Nursing Practice* 9 2: 37-47.

Emblem JD and Halstead L (1993): Spiritual needs and interventions: comparing the views of patients, nurses and chaplains. *Clinical Nurse Specialist* 7 4: 175-182.

Evans D (1993): *Spirituality and Human Nature*. New York: State University of New York.

Hall C and Lanig H (1993): Spiritual caring behaviours as reported by Christian nurses. *Western Journal of Nursing Research* 15 6: 730-741.

Harrington A (1995): Spiritual care: what does it mean to RNs? *Australian Journal of Advanced Nursing* 12 4: 5-13.

Kim MJ, McFarland GK, McLane AM (eds) (1987) *Pocket Guide to Nursing Diagnosis* (2nd edn). St Louis: CV Mosby.

Kübler-Ross E (1975): *Death, the Final Stage of Growth.* New Jersey: Prentice Hall.

MacKinlay E (1996): Meeting the spiritual needs of the elderly. *Spirituality in Nursing Practice.* Papers from a conference held on 27 March 1996 at The Swiss Grand Hotel, Bondi, Australia. Melbourne: Ausmed Publications.

Macrae J (1995): Nightingale's spiritual philosophy and its significance for modern nursing. *IMAGE: Journal of Nursing Scholarship* 27 1, Spring.

Meleis A (1991): *Theoretical Nursing: Development and Progress.* Philadelphia: JB Lippincott Company.

Merton T (1960): *Spiritual Direction and Meditation.*

Collegeville, Minnesota: Liturgical Press.

Narayanasamy A (1993): Nurses' awareness and educational preparation in meeting their patients' spiritual needs. *Nurse Education Today* 13: 196-201.

Oldnall A (1995): On the absence of spirituality in nursing theories and models. *Journal of Advanced Nursing* 21: 417-418.

Parse RR (1987): *Nursing Science: Major Paradigms, Theories and Critiques.* Philadelphia: WB Saunders Company.

Patience A (1991): Softening the hard culture. *Mental Health in Australia* 3 3: 29-35.

Reed PG (1992): An emerging paradigm for the investigation of spirituality in nursing. *Research in Nursing and Health* 15: 349-357.

Ross LA (1994): Spiritual aspects of nursing. *Journal of Advanced Nursing* 19: 439-447.

Smith SG (1988): *The Concept of the Spiritual: An Essay in First Philosophy.* Philadelphia: Temple Press.

Stiles MK (1994): The shining stranger: Application of the phenomenological method in the investigation of the nurse–family spiritual relationship. *Cancer Nursing* 17 1 18-26.

Streubert HJ and Carpenter DR (1995): *Qualitative Research in Nursing: Advancing the Humanistic Imperative.* Philadelphia: JB Lippincott Company.

Vaughan F (1995): *Shadows of the Sacred: Seeing through Spiritual Illusions.* Wheaton: Quest Books.

Williams RM (1970): *American Society: A Sociological Interpretation* (2nd edn). New York: Knopf.

OTHER READING

Carson VB (1989): *Spiritual Dimensions of Nursing Practice.* Philadelphia: WB Saunders Company.

Mitchell ML (1989): Spirituality in psychiatric/mental health nursing. In: Birckhead L (ed.) *Psychiatric Mental Health Nursing: The Therapeutic Use of Self.* Philadelphia: JB Lippincott Company.

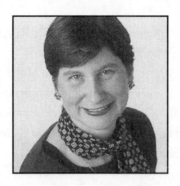

JANE HALL
RN, Midwife, BAppSci(AdvNursEd), MEd, FRCNA, FACM

Jane is a nurse-midwife and healer. She has a private practice and consultancy in healing and education. She is a teacher and practitioner of Therapeutic Touch and a practitioner of Healing Touch and Kinesiology.

Jane has extensive experience in women's health, especially birthing. She also has a background in administration as a senior nursing adviser in the Victorian Health Department in Australia. She was a senior lecturer at the Australian Catholic University and continues to guest lecture at several universities. Jane is also a member of the inaugural Nurses Board of Victoria.

Jane conducts seminars centred around personal development for mothers, nurses, midwives and other healers, including workshops exploring the wounded healer, in both Sydney and Melbourne. She uses many innovative and inspiring approaches to nurture, enrich and enliven participants. She has recently established Healing Connections, in partnership with Sue Dawson, which aims to facilitate the teaching and integration of Therapeutic Touch in the health care system.

Chapter 2

NURSES AS WOUNDED HEALERS

INTRODUCTION: SPIRITUALITY AS NURSING BUSINESS

Illness, birth and death are all times when our ordinary reality is disrupted, and we are confronted with the deeper and sometimes darker (or brighter) aspects of ourselves. The security of the everyday world is called into question and we visit anew the profound and mysterious questions of vulnerability, pain, suffering, creation and death. Even nonserious incidents can cause rethinking of purpose and direction as they interrupt the flow of our lives.

Healing therefore encompasses more than cure or treatment, more than nurture; it involves making 'more whole'. As such it is a process of finding the transforming possibilities in the experience. This requires making sense out of the experience, finding meaning, and placing the experience within one's belief system and life. This involves the soul, that is the deeper parts of self beyond everyday consciousness which seek to deepen experience. The aspect of self called spirit — the connection with the greater, the wider, that which is within yet beyond self — is an inherent part of this soul work. As Carson (1989) identifies, spirituality can be defined in a multitude of ways.

For the purposes of this chapter, spirituality will be taken to relate to both soul and spirit, that is to the essence of who we are, which is not separate from but pervades and unifies body, mind and emotion (Carson, 1989). Our spirituality involves our connection to that which is beyond self, whether universal values or the divine, as well as connection to nature and to other people who, as Carson (1989) points out, provide love, meaning and purpose in life. For some there is a framework for their spirituality in the form of a belief system, or religion, however, the extent to which this is helpful may depend upon their own spiritual path and understanding. Seen from the perspective of this chapter, as outlined above, spirituality cannot be set apart in a church or temple, but is present in the everyday reality of disrupted or changed body functions, destabilised emotions, disrupted thought patterns and lives changed or torn apart.

Nurses and midwives accompany people through these life experiences. We engage in the process of healing as we assist people to make the extraordinary ordinary and to find the meaning and possibility inherent in their experience (Benner, 1984; Benner and Wrubel, 1989; Taylor, 1994, 1995). Nurses and midwives are with people in the quiet and private places of bath and birth, and in the dark reaches of the night. We are present at those times and places when the cry of soul and spirit can be heard over the bustle of life. So, whether we admit it or not, spirituality is nursing business. We are involved in clients' spirituality whenever we practise and our own spirituality is affected. If we wish to facilitate healing of the whole person then we must consciously engage in the spiritual aspect of ourselves and those for whom we care. Visiting the wisdom of ancient and traditional cultures gives us insight into the healer for whom spirituality is an integral part of life.

This chapter presents the notion of the wounded healer as a pattern for the preparation of a healer who is equipped to work with the whole person, body, mind, emotion and soul/spirit.

THE WOUNDED HEALER: A PATTERN FOR HEALERS

Mythology contains the sacred truths of a culture in the form of story. Deep wisdom about the human condition, including what it is to be involved in healing, is expressed in stories of divine and special beings. Exploration of these stories results in understandings about how we should approach our lives and our practice as healers. The notion of the wounded healer can be found in the mythology of numerous cultures as well as in ancient healing traditions and in modern medicine in the area of transpersonal psychology. Examination of the many and varied forms it has taken has led to the identification of a pattern which can be used for the preparation and ongoing development of healers of any type and in any culture (Hall, 1994). The particular value of the notion of the wounded healer is that it originates from cultures which have tended to a more holistic view of what it is to be human and of the healing process, that is, where spirituality is recognised as an integral part of healing.

The pattern of the wounded healer is most clearly exemplified in the 'great' stories of Aesclepius the Greek god of medicine, in Christ and in the Buddha. These archetypal wounded healers, who were both divine and human, were wounded in body, soul and spirit and as members of a community. They experienced deep wounding which involved not only physical and emotional distress, but spiritual wounding through encounters with the dark and demonic (for instance, the Buddha's encounter with the demon Mara) and severance from their source of meaning, that is from higher self or spirit. For Aesclepius this took the form of death by the hand of the great god, Zeus (Houston, 1987; Hall, 1994, 1996).

After the initial wounding each healer undertook a journey which involved trial and suffering. In the case of Christ, the journey also involved underworld time, a place which represents the soul. Eventually, through assistance from the higher self or spirit, the journey was completed and healing in the form of transformation to the highest state of being was experienced. From this basis, as divine or enlightened beings, they went on to heal many others (Hall, 1994, 1996).

The core feature in these great stories is that the experience of wounding was followed by the experience of healing. Healers must come to know and experience both their wounding — which may take many forms including the experience of vulnerability, pain, hurt, suffering or betrayal — and the healing of their wounds. Furthermore, the process involves all aspects of self — body, mind, emotion, soul and spirit — in connection with that which is outside and beyond self. Healing does not happen in isolation.

Ancient healing traditions, such as the shamanic healing of indigenous peoples (including the Australian Aborigines and the native Americans), the Ayurvedic medicine of India and the Unani medicine of Islamic cultures, have understood this and translated such wisdom into processes for the preparation and ongoing development of their healers. They recognise the significance of the 'call to healing' that is the reason why a person chooses to become a healer. The call is often through personal trauma, which must be dealt with to free the person for healing. The message for modern healers is that this and other wounds should not be denied or hidden, for they have great value. The process of acknowledging and dealing with wounds can release considerable healing 'power'. From this perspective our wounds become sacred (Hall, 1996).

The shaman's preparation involves a complex and arduous process with deep wounding from physical to spiritual levels. This provides preparation for the deeply spiritual nature of shamanic work. The shaman experiences this journey many times, for as a human healer, the development of wholeness is an ongoing part of life (Hall, 1994). Other healing systems such as Ayurveda are not necessarily as dramatic, showing that a healer's preparation and journey can take the form of the gradual development of wisdom gained through the experience of life and healing. For many traditional healing systems preparation of healers is aimed at the development of personal characteristics such as compassion, moral/ethical maturity and the ability to relate to people. This goes hand in hand with the acquisition of the specific knowledge and skills required for healing practice. Modern education for healing tends to ignore the development of the healer's character and generally pays little if any attention to spirituality.

The shaman and other traditional healers may seem very far removed from our experience as modern healers for we have split the healing function so that different professions are 'experts' on different parts of the person. Spirituality is seen as the province of the chaplain or pastoral care worker and perhaps the psychologist. However, nurses cross these boundaries for we are with the person in the reality of their lived experience. We tend their bodies and relate to their everyday, ordinary consciousness of thought and feeling. In dealing with the most profound life experiences of illness, birth and death, we are also involved in shamanic-like situations for, as Sandford (1977) argues, anything which causes disruption of everyday consciousness and provides the opportunity for awareness at deeper levels constitutes a shamanic experience or journey of the soul, with its need for spiritual support and guidance. This requires a person who is equipped to guide the other on their journey, that is, someone who has taken the journey, a wounded healer. As these pre-modern cultures knew, dealing with such life experiences can be very powerful and can demand much from the healer. Healers themselves require guidance and support.

In summary, the core elements of the pattern of the wounded healer are a call to healing of some kind, which often involves wounding — a process of self-awareness, of becoming aware of one's wounds, and of exploring them. There is a journey towards healing which involves the whole self (body, mind, emotion, soul and spirit), a letting go of cherished views of self and patterns of thought (disinte-gration) and a process of growth (reintegration), of putting back together in a new form. Healing involves a movement towards wholeness and achieving greater balance, coming into 'right' relationship with all parts of self so that transfor-mation, creativity and self-actualisation can occur (Artress, 1995; Hall, 1994, 1996; Krieger, 1997; Quinn, 1989). Through this path the person becomes a wounded healer, equipped to reach out to others in a relationship charac-terised by love and compassion, and so assist the other on the journey from wounding to healing.

USING THE PATTERN OF THE WOUNDED HEALER FOR NURSING: CONSIDERING WOUNDEDNESS

Examination of nursing literature reveals many dimensions of woundedness for nurses which can be related to the concepts of power, invisibility, knowledge, life experiences, work environments and the embodied self (Hall, 1994). The first step in using the pattern of the wounded healer is to recognise and explore the 'wounds' of nurses. The wisdom expressed in stories related to the wounded healer gives some pointers as to how this may be approached.

Just as wounding and healing appear together in mythology — for example, many deities such as the Babylonian goddess Ishtar (Jayne, 1925) could both wound and heal — so should modern healers consider their wounds in tandem with their healing. For instance, there is particular emphasis in nursing literature on the powerlessness of nurses and its end results, such as horizontal violence (Duffy, 1995). Concentration on this form of woundedness can result in a sense of paralysis, a loss of hope and meaning. Recognising that nurses' very lack of power has a healing aspect (for it brings us close to our clients and lays the groundwork for a healing relationship based on equality and shared power) provides an entirely different viewpoint (Oakley, 1986; Hall, 1994; Hall, Miller and Seibold, 1997). From this perspective, healing for nurses may well be that they would not always seek power just by climbing the hierarchy. Rather, nurses may work for the power which Benner (1984) and Street (1992) describe as growing out of a strong commitment to clients and a caring therapeutic relationship.

Telephus was a warrior in the Trojan wars who could only be healed by the rust from the spear which wounded him (Kerenyi, 1959). This story suggests that the wound provides clues to its own healing and so emphasises the value of nurses exploring and listening to their wounds. Much of what nurses do is hidden for we deal with aspects of body, self and life which are private, and we act to make the 'extraordinary' experiences of ill health 'ordinary' (Taylor, 1994, 1995). Nurses are wounded by the invisibility and lack of recognition that results. One clue to healing contained in this wound is that nurses are visible and valued by those who have received care. As the midwives in New Zealand have done, nurses might harness this knowledge, which has come out of a healing relationship, and work in partnership with their clients to gain improvements in health care as well as recognition for themselves (Guilliland and Pairman, 1995).

Indian mythology indicates that woundedness and healing should be viewed as opposite polarities, existing in dynamic balance within a person and a healing relationship (Hall, 1996). Undue emphasis on either polarity will lead to a lack of balance. In terms of nurses' woundedness in relation to knowledge, nursing education has tended to focus on the intellectual and skill-based aspects of the discipline while neglecting aspects such as self-awareness, personal growth and the ability to use self therapeutically. Balance could be provided in numerous ways such as the inclusion of nursing literature dealing with caring and healing theory. At present nurses can and do seek out balance through their own studies and the pursuit of such adjuncts to practice as those complementary therapies (for example, massage) which enhance the healing relationship. As the pattern of the wounded healer demonstrates, a balanced approach to education requires the ongoing support and guidance of mentors and teachers who themselves are wounded healers.

Nurses face many demands as they work with people in the midst of their suffering, trauma and also joy. Paradoxically when nurses engage in healing it means being involved, coming even closer to clients' pain, as well as to their happiness. This increases nurses' vulnerability (Gadow, 1980, 1989). What is more, nurses bring their own life experiences of woundedness including, for this mainly female population, the pressures of home and family, grief, loss of love and, for one in ten women, abuse (Hall, 1996; McMurray and Moore, 1994). They bring these wounds to an environment which is largely unsupportive and often damaging (Hall, 1994, 1996). As Street (1992) identified in her ethnographic study of nursing, separateness from the support of colleagues is endemic within nursing. Nurses are taught to hide their personal pain, to 'cope' with anything. This is clearly revealed in a survey of nurses who experienced traumatic events. A number of those who responded had internalised their trauma after receiving strong messages from colleagues and management to keep quiet (Buyssen, 1996).

Furthermore, Menzies (1961) has argued that the demands of nursing activate past wounds, especially those in childhood, and that these result in extensive social defence mechanisms which have become deeply embedded in nursing culture. It is small wonder that nurses have developed deeply embodied and largely unconscious distancing and defence mechanisms for self-protection (Hall, 1994). Ironically these defences cause further damage for they separate nurses from their source of meaning, from much which can offer healing, that is, their inner selves, their clients, and each other.

Woundedness and its associated defences inevitably affect the healing relationship for, in various ways, woundedness acts to reduce connectedness. Much of the modern literature on the wounded healer is concerned with the consequences of wounding, that, is of healers failing to take the journey from wounding to healing (Adler, 1984; Guggenbuhl-Craig, 1971; Groesbeck, 1975; Miller and Baldwin, 1987; Remen et al., 1985; Zigmond, 1984). The results may range from simply not having enough energy for the deeper aspects of healing to nurses actively undermining a client's sense of self and healing ability through the misuse of power. At best the healing relationship lacks effectiveness and clients struggle to heal with reduced help. At worst clients are actively harmed by the experience of health care. Nurses are also negatively affected and can experience stress, burnout and failure to heal self. In the end the great and deep wound of betrayal is experienced where clients are damaged by those from whom they seek care, and nurses wound each other in spirals of horizontal violence (Hall, 1994, 1997).

While nurses' wounding occurs on many levels from the societal to the personal and the physical it is, in the end, a spiritual issue. Carson (1989) points out the similarities between burnout (as described in nursing literature) and spiritual stress. Nurses in the process of burning out experience loss of meaning with accompanying fear, guilt, depression and boredom. They suffer from apathy, stagnation and loss of hope. The result is withdrawal and isolation from others. If nurses are to attend to their clients' spiritual needs it is imperative they attend to their own spirituality, that is, to their wounding and its healing.

THE JOURNEY TO HEALING

The heart of spirituality in nursing is to be found in a healing relationship, which involves connection at a human-to-human level, caring and compassion, trust and respect for human dignity. This can be established as nurses provide physical care, and through listening to their clients and their colleagues in the sharing of everyday practice. As Watson (1988) has identified in her description of a caring–healing consciousness, the healing effects of nursing care cross the boundaries of space and time. For example, an understanding word at the right moment can assist a person to recover as it is remembered over days, weeks or years. This requires quality of time where there is attention, and the nurse is fully 'present', rather than quantity of time. Spiritual care can therefore be an inherent part of nursing practice rather than an additional extra to be provided 'when time allows'. The factors that wound nurses act in various ways to interrupt the healing relationship. Dealing with wounds opens the doors to nurses' own healing and to their ability to attend to another's spirituality on a day-to-day basis.

It is in the healing relationship that nurses and other healers find some of their healing (Adler, 1984; Miller and Baldwin, 1987; Remen et al., 1985). Studies by Swanson (1990) and Montgomery (1991) indicate that nurses who are able to resist burnout and to care in the presence of demanding situations are those who can access the therapeutic relationship. Montgomery (1991) and Benner (1991) both argue that it is the experience of caring which leads to confidence, self-esteem and energy and which protects from burnout. Montgomery (1991) found that when this is combined with wider values and beliefs (that is, connected to the spiritual aspects of being) burnout can be avoided. It is engagement with the other which enriches, protects and empowers the healer (Hall, 1994, 1997).

The process of nursing is therefore part of nurses' spirituality. The feeding of the soul which comes from the tenderness of caring and the connection with clients in the healing relationship leads us to the paradox that our spirituality supports our practice and our practice feeds our spirituality. In her book *Living the Therapeutic Touch* the nurse–healer Dolores Krieger (1979) describes this process. She states: 'the reality of the healing act can activate compelling life affirmative drives in those who heal'. She describes such nurses as follows:

> They are responsive to creativity, spontaneity, expressiveness and idiosyncracity in self and in others. They sense meaningfulness in life because they have touched the more subtle reaches of its nature during their peak experiences of helping others (Krieger, 1979:16).

Krieger (1993) also identifies that pursuit of healing arts (or therapies) such as Therapeutic Touch can lead to personal growth. She has since completed a book devoted to the process of undertaking inner work (Krieger, 1997).

Healing for nurses with regard to their professional lives and activities can therefore include pursuit of those models of care (such as team midwifery or primary nursing) and areas of practice (including appropriate healing therapies) which facilitate development of the nurse–client relationship. Contact with colleagues and mentors who are concerned with providing holistic care and a focus on education that supports healing practice are also essential. The process of healing also requires personal work, which sustains professional practice.

WALKING THE LABYRINTH: A PATH TO HEALING

There are many avenues for nurses to take to assist them in exploring their own wounding and healing. Choices should be based on personal preference, as well as readiness to attend to certain aspects of self. There is no need to face up to all one's woundedness at once! However, it is important to commence the journey, one that lasts a lifetime, and as time passes matters that require attention will become clear. Many spiritual disciplines offer guidelines for this process. In this chapter the ancient archetypal symbol of the labyrinth will be used to provide a template to guide nurses as they attend to their own healing.

The labyrinth is a walking meditation based on a complex spiral form. The path inwards to the centre is followed, during which a process of letting go occurs. The centre provides a quiet space for contemplation and insight. The path outward mirrors the inward way. The person walks back into everyday life strengthened and empowered (Artress, 1995).

As Lawler (1991) identified, nurses deal with bodies continually. Just as this is a walking meditation involving the body, so should the journey for nurses include attention to their own bodies. Nurses need to listen to the messages of their bodies, which also contain many defences. For instance, some nurses are quite happy to touch clients but are very uncomfortable about being touched themselves (Hall, unpublished student evaluations, 1993). Common ailments such as back pain may have a physical cause but can reflect feelings of lack of support and a sense of insecurity (Hay, 1984; Myss, 1996). Therapies such as yoga and Feldenkrais, which tend the body and connect it to the rest of self, may be useful.

The walk inwards allows reflection on, then letting go of, everyday concerns. This translates into recognising and exploring wounds using processes such as those described previously. However, as Myss (1996) points out, there is a danger of becoming attached to one's wounds, of being stuck in the journey to healing rather than reaching the end point and letting the wound go. It must also be recognised that, at some stage, confronting wounds and reaching for healing involves facing up to the darker side of self, the 'shadow' — to confronting anger and guilt, fear, the need for power and the ability to blame others. At some level and in some way it is necessary to let go of a dearly held perspective on self and, even as the shamans did, to experience disintegration (Hall, 1997). The path inwards is a cleansing and quietening process which prepares for reaching the centre (Artress, 1995:67).

The centre of the labyrinth is the place of illumination. It represents the going to the centre of self and accessing the wisdom which lies within. This can involve just being still, contemplating nature or using various forms of meditation. Healing at the deepest level comes from this realm, this is the place of 'knowing' which is beyond the intellect, the seat of intuition and insight, it is the place of meeting with the divine.

Illumination also comes from beyond self. This may occur through connection with the divine in stillness or prayer or through connection to other sources of wisdom. For instance, accessing literature on nursing, and on healing, especially stories of other wounded healers such as Ian Gawler (1984), Oliver Sacks (1991), Tony Moore (1991) and Norman Cousins (1979), can be helpful.

The spiritual guidance, deep knowledge and wisdom, and the rituals and symbols inherent in belief systems can also be utilised. For instance, nurses could consider actually walking a labyrinth, or accessing the many and varied short courses, seminars and groups available in the community. Courses that combine transpersonal psychology and spirituality, for example, to explore the wounded-healer concept can provide profound insights. It may be useful to access various tools to assist in gaining insight; processes such as keeping a journal and reflecting on self as well as practice are very valuable. Visualisation, imagery, art, music or dance can enrich the journey and be the source of much joy.

The last and vital step involves walking out of the labyrinth, which is symbolic of reconnecting with the personal and professional world. Nouwen (1972) suggests that the process of finding the light and dark inside of self involves making space for the entry of the spirit, and through this to connection with the frailty of the human condition. The wound becomes the training ground for the development of compassion and allows healing to be completed in reaching out to connect with others, through the shared experience of the journey. The healer is strengthened, energised and empowered through this process (Artress, 1995).

The labyrinth represents 'sacred space' a place where wounds are honoured and respected, and where fear and vulnerability can be acknowledged. Appropriate support people, such as professional mentors, a spiritual director, friends and family can provide this space. The setting aside of a sacred space at home, which is private and inviolate, or visiting a special place such as a natural environment, can offer healing to the spirit.

Nurses can take the wisdom, knowledge and healing techniques obtained through their own healing journey back out into the world for use in practice. Just as the labyrinth can be walked many times, so should nurses walk the journey from wounding to healing, even on a daily basis, emerging each time with new strength and healing energy for themselves and others.

CONCLUSION: THE NURSE AS WOUNDED HEALER

Nurses as wounded healers are distinguished by personal characteristics and an ability to enter into healing relationships. They appear less ego-driven, able to set aside their own need to succeed, able to centre on the client. As Montgomery (1991) says, connection with the client is the primary goal of such nurses; other goals such as solving problems derive from the healing relationship. Krieger (1993) says that this centredness involves respect for an individual's dynamic and enables full engagement of the nurse's energies with the intent of helping the client. This paves the way for the acquisition of the deeper and intuitive knowledge and understanding which is part of spirituality.

Through the experience of their own journey from wounding to healing nurses can develop knowledge and skills in dealing with the deeper aspects of self and in enhancing the process of finding meaning in experience, that is, in the spiritual aspects of healing. The recognition of mutual woundedness acts as connection in the healing relationship and prevents the assumption of distance and superiority. As Taylor (1995) says, this involves meeting on the grounds of common humanity. Inherent in this relationship is the caring love and compassion which flows out of the healer's personal growth. Sheila Mitchie (1996), a nurse in independent practice, describes being a wounded healer as follows:

> . . . through our wounding and continual healing we become aware of our connectedness to all life. There is no separation, there are no them and us, there is only all of us irrevocably bound together, searching for love. As we express God's love more deeply and openly, those who are touched by our presence discover a safe sacred place where they are accepted with respect and understanding, a place filled with love where they can reveal their vulnerability and wounding and where healing can begin. (Mitchie, 1996:60)

In summary, the notion of the wounded healer offers individual nurses and the nursing profession a pattern which may be used not only for healing practice but for their own self-knowledge, creativity, and transformation. This is a sacred process in a secular society; it requires both commitment and courage, while offering fulfilment and a guiding vision for nursing and healing in the next millennium.

REFERENCES

Adler G (1984): Regarding the wounded healer. *British Journal of Holistic Medicine* 1: 131-132.

Artress L (1995): *Walking a Sacred Path*: Rediscovering the labyrinth as a spiritual tool. New York: Riverhead Books.

Benner P (1984): *From Novice to Expert*: Excellence and power in clinical nursing practice. Menlo Park, California: Addison Wesley.

Benner P (1991): The role of experience, narrative and community in skilled ethical deportment. *Advances in Nursing Science* 14 2: 1-21.

Benner P and Wrubel J (1989): *The Primacy of Caring*. Menlo Park, California: Addison Wesley.

Buyssen H (1996): *Traumatic Experiences of Nurses*: When your profession becomes a nightmare. London: Jessica Kingsley Publishers.

Carson VB (1989): *Spiritual Dimensions of Nursing Practice*. Philadelphia: WB Saunders.

Cousins N (1979): *Anatomy of an Illness*. New York: Bantam.

Duffy E (1995): Horizontal violence: a conundrum for nursing. *Collegian* 2 2: 5-17.

Gadow S (1980): Existential advocacy: philosophical foundation of nursing. In: Spicker SF (ed.): *Nursing: Images and Ideals*. Open dialogue with the humanities. New York: Springer, pp. 79-99.

Gadow S (1989): Clinical subjectivity: advocacy with silent patients. *Nursing Clinics of North America* 24 2: 535-541.

Gawler I (1984): *You Can Conquer Cancer*. Melbourne: Hill of Content.

Groesbeck CJ (1975): The archetypal image of the wounded healer. *Journal of Analytical Psychology* 20 1: 122-145.

Guggenbuhl-Craig A (1971): *Power in the Helping Professions*. Dallas: Spring.

Guilliland K and Pairman S (1995): The Midwifery Partnership: A Model for Practice. Monograph Series 95/1. Wellington, New Zealand: Department of Nursing and Midwifery, Victoria University.

Hall (1993): Unpublished student evaluations.

Hall JS (1994): Nurses as wounded-healers. Unpublished Masters Thesis. Bundoora, Melbourne, Australia: La Trobe University.

Hall JS (1996): Challenges to caring: Nurses as wounded-healers. Part A. *Australian Journal of Holistic Nursing* 3 2: 12-18.

Hall JS (1997): Nurses as wounded-healers: The journey to healing the person and profession. Part B. *Australian Journal of Holistic Nursing* 4 1: 11-16.

Hall JS, Miller M, Seibold C (1997): Truth or fiction? Partnership in labour: dealing with pain. Proceedings of the Australian College of Midwives Inc. 10th Biennial Conference. Melbourne, 16-18 April.

Houston J (1987): *Search for the Beloved*: Journeys in Mythology and Sacred Psychology. New York: Jeremy P. Tarcher.

Jayne WA (1925): *The Healing Gods of Ancient Civilisations*. New Haven: Yale University Press.

Kerenyi C (1959): *Asklepios: Archetypal Image of the Physicians Existence*. Trans. R Manheim. New York: Pantheon.

Krieger D (1979): *Living the Therapeutic Touch: Healing as a Lifestyle*. New York: Dodd Mead.

Krieger D (1993): *Accepting Your Power to Heal: The Personal Practice of Therapeutic Touch*. Sante Fe: Bear and Co.

Krieger D (1997): *Therapeutic Touch: Inner Workbook*. Sante Fe: Bear and Co.

Lawler J (1991): *Behind the Screens: Nursing, Somology and the Problem of the Body*. Melbourne: Churchill Livingstone.

McMurray A and Moore K (1994): Domestic violence: Are we listening? Do we see? *Australian Journal of Advanced Nursing* 12 1: 23-26.

Menzies I (1961): *The Functioning of Social Systems as a Defence Against Anxiety: A Report of a Study of Nursing Service of a General Hospital*. London: Tavistock.

Miller GD and Baldwin DC (1987): Implications of the wounded healer paradigm for the use of self in therapy. *Journal of Psychotherapy and the Family* 3 1: 139-151.

Mitchie, S. (1995): The holistic healer is the wounded-healer. *Golden Age* p.60.

Moore T (1991): *Cry of the Damaged Man: A Personal Journey of Recovery*. Sydney: Picador.

Montgomery CL (1991): The care-giving relationship: parad-oxical and transcendent aspects. *Journal of Trans-personal Psychology* 23 2: 91-103.

Myss C (1996): *Anatomy of the Spirit: The Seven Stages of Power and Healing*. New York: Bantam.

Nouwen HJM (1972): *The Wounded Healer* — ministry in contemporary society. New York: Doubleday and Co. Inc.

Oakley A (1986): *Telling the Truth about Jerusalem*. Oxford: Basil Blackwell.

Quinn J (1989): Healing, whole-ness and the haelen effect. *Nursing and Health Care* 10 10: 553-556.

Remen N, May R, Young D and Berland W (1985): The wounded healer. *Saybrook Review* 5 1: 84-93.

Sacks O (1991): *A Leg To Stand On*. London: Picador.

Sandford S (1977): *Healing and Wholeness*. New York: Paulist Press.

Street A (1992): *Inside Nursing: A Critical Ethnography of Clinical Nursing Practice*. Albany: University of New York Press.

Swanson KM (1990): Providing care in the NICU: Sometimes an act of love. *Advances in Nursing Science* 13 1: 60-73.

Taylor B (1994): *Being Human: Ordinariness in Nursing*. Melbourne: Churchill Livingstone.

Taylor B (1995): Nursing as healing work. *Contemporary Nurse* 4: 100-106.

Watson J (1988): New dimensions of human caring theory. *Nursing Science Quarterly*. 1 4: 175-181.

Zigmond D (1984): Physician heal thyself: the paradox of the wounded healer. *British Journal of Holistic Medicine* 1: 63-71.

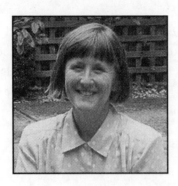

LINDA WALTER
RN

In the 1960s Linda Walter trained as a nurse at Royal Children's Hospital in Melbourne and at Royal Melbourne Hospital. She nursed in Geelong, Australia, and the UK before marrying and raising a family.

For the past fifteen years she has trained and worked in hospital pastoral care and counselling. She is active in the Christian feminist movement and in 1989 she co-authored, with Janet Nelson, a book on feminism and Christianity called *Women of Spirit*, published by St Mark's National Theological Centre in Canberra. Linda now lectures in palliative care, and counsels from her home in Melbourne.

Chapter 3

THE PATIENT NURSE

It is not possible to define spirituality neatly. The presence and activity of the Spirit is glimpsed within an individual life and in the life we see happening around us in the world. These glimpses are recognised because of their effects: a heightened awareness; a sense of being more alive (both to pain and pleasure); the experience of being more deeply connected to one's self and to surroundings (to people, to the natural world, to things); a felt understanding of a 'presence' which is more, and other, than the sum of the parts, a presence which calls forth some response.

We are told that the Spirit blows where it wills. In the things of the Spirit we find ourselves in the realm of surprise and wonder and uncertainty. Is 'spirituality', then, how we name our struggle to define what must always elude definition? A rough word, clumsy but necessary, in a time of disillusionment with organised religions? A democratic word that allows everybody to ponder and honour his or her own experiences of the mystery at the heart of human existence?

Nursing and spirituality come together in my own life in a particularly vivid way. My years of work as both nurse and chaplain turn on my experience as patient. What I discovered in that time of serious illness many years ago changed me.

I was a nurse and thought I knew all I needed to know about hospitals and illness. I didn't. I was a woman of faith and thought I knew what I needed to know about prayer and spirituality. I didn't. The discoveries that changed me I now understand were to do with power and powerlessness. My gratitude for my recovery at the hands of skilled surgical and nursing staff is enormous. But my most vivid and precious memory, still, twenty years later, is of a very ordinary moment that held my body and spirit together when I feared I had lost both. Two nurses washed me. They were efficient and thorough. It was a busy ward. But they knew what they were doing and they did it with utmost tenderness. They washed every inch of me, and though I was powerless and vulnerable, they left me feeling neither overpowered nor patronised. I felt their respect for me. I knew they were *seeing* me. They said very little but they called me by my name. I knew they were seeing *me*. They had ministered to my body and my soul and to the life-giving connection between them which is what I have come to understand spirituality to be.

These two nurses made me proud of my chosen profession and determined never to despise the most simple aspects of bedside nursing care. A back injury took me out of nursing and a love of listening led me into chaplaincy. It is during the past fifteen years' pastoral counselling, mostly in a cancer hospital, that I have, through experience and reflection, gleaned the insights offered in this chapter. As a pastoral counsellor I worked with patients undergoing treatment, with patients and relatives dealing with the transition from active treatment to palliation, and with staff throughout the hospital. I offered bereavement support to grieving relatives — both individually and in groups — and lectured on loss and grief to postgraduate nurses, hospice workers and medical students.

Over the years it has become very evident to me that many health workers long to find a more simple openness in dealing with the realities of life and death. Most health professionals find difficulty in balancing the two realities: this patient may get better and live/this patient may deteriorate and die. They understand the importance of hopefulness in staff and patients if treatments are to be successful. However, maintaining a hopeful attitude too often is interpreted as 'having to be positive at all costs'. Such a 'positive' stance can become a heavy burden on everyone concerned and can make honest communications and democratic choices concerning management of the disease very difficult for patients and relatives as well as for staff. This in turn can create a climate of half-truths and evasions, or make it seem that a kind of brutal clinical honesty is the only alternative. When patient and staff get caught up in a fiercely hopeful (almost omnipotent) optimism, there is an increased need to defend against the only apparent alternative, that is, a hopeless (powerless) pessimism. It is here that the temptation to withhold information from the patient is probably strongest, a temptation that stems from the nurse's refusal to feel her/his own powerlessness. To hold the facts of illness and treatment and the possibilities of life and death in creative and fluid tension, without splitting into either optimism or pessimism, is not easy. Nurses are in a particularly crucial position to create a working environment where such holding can happen.

As both nurse and chaplain, I have learnt much from staff and patients and their families. But, ironically, I have learnt most from the relatives and loved ones who come after a death for bereavement counselling — either in groups or individually. Bereavement counselling has been another lesson in powerlessness. The only thing that would make a grieving person 'better' is to bring back the dead person. The one thing that might be expected to gratify me, the helper, is to see the grieving person happy. We, the grieving one and the helping one, are powerless to please one another — to heal or to appear healed. So what has this sort of powerlessness taught me about power? How might it help us to think of our own use or abuse of power in the care of patients? And what has power got to do with nurses and spirituality?

It seems to me the clue is that after the patient dies everyone stops pretending. The truth is undeniable and the 'tasks of healthy grieving' (in the words of William Worden, 1983) are to accept this hard fact of death, to lean into the pain of the loss and to begin to adjust to a life without that person, learning eventually to take the risk of trusting life and of opening to love again. This work of grief is hard, lonely, painful work and it takes commitment and patience and real courage over a long period of time.

Whether we are bereavement counsellors, nurses, or helpers in any profession, we cannot effect this process. At best we can encourage it by our respectful attention and patient companionship. It is the grieving person herself who must slog a path through the dark valley, as anyone who has grieved a loved one will know well. Some describe it as a dark valley, others say grief is a roller-coaster ride: dizzying and sickening. I have heard the experience of bereavement called a 'grief-storm', like being alone at sea in a tiny boat, at times contending with the terror of unpredictable waves and winds, at times becalmed in a dense fog, exposed, without bearings. No wonder as onlookers we cannot bear what we see, nor the helplessness we feel. No wonder many of us turn away — or try to rescue. The 'helping professions', by definition, find such helplessness in the face of pain particularly hard to bear. Yet, if it is true that one of the tasks of healthy grieving is to experience the pain of the loss, then our attempts to rescue and protect the griever from the pain only make it worse in the end — harder and longer.

When I originally began this bereavement work it was with the understanding that I was there to offer support to grieving people through listening to those who came to me, and through facilitating bereavement support groups. I was there to help people 'cope', to help them get back to some sort of stability where life was bearable again. This is still a worthwhile aim of bereavement support. But I have seen something more remarkable happening in this work. I have seen some people become empowered through their grieving. When a person is not stopped from expressing feelings of utter despair, when he is encouraged to voice how it really is for him in all its blackness and hopelessness, when she is able to admit to and give vent to anger and rage, then there can come a point when, in the midst of despair, hope is engendered of itself. And within this hopefulness lies a tender, resilient power. It is not something which group leaders or counsellors can instil. It is intrinsic in the grieving person and is born out of the struggle to be true to the full experience of grief. The courage to face despair and to wait within it is not easily found. There are many people who manage to find all the love and support they need within their own circle of family and friends. For some, though, this is simply not the case and they may need to look for support — either one to one, or in the company of strangers who share a similar grief. When grieving people come together in a group they can find a collective courage which literally encourages each individual member to face his own despair.

A social worker with whom I have led these bereavement groups became excited when I spoke with her of empowerment as the possible outcome of bereavement support. She had sensed the emergence of hope but had not articulated it for herself or to me, being wary of overstatement and having a healthy resistance to religious language. But, named or unnamed, this is what can happen. We did not speak of hope. Hope, I have discovered, is not a commodity or an attitude that can be given. Nor for that matter can it be taken away. Hope is not the same thing as optimism. Being hopeful is deeper than being determined to 'stay positive'. This is because mature hope is always grounded in the facts: it struggles to hold onto both 'positive' and 'negative' aspects of the truth of the situation. Grieving can only begin when the fact of loss has registered. So, though hope is not a thing that can be 'given' or 'taken away', it cannot emerge where there is neither openness nor honesty. We begin to see that this kind of mature hope simply cannot be formed in a climate of half-truths and evasions. This is what I have learned from bereavement counselling and I believe it has implications for nurses in their dealings with patients and families right from the first moment of contact with one another.

It would seem that our well-meaning efforts to protect patients and relatives from painful information during diagnosis, treatments, results of tests, reviews of treatment options, prognosis, and the transition from radical treatment to palliative care and pain control are often ultimately not truly helpful to the patient. These protective measures — often so subtle that we do not realise we are using them — can prevent the true reality from being faced. Sometimes the information is truthfully given but the interpretations of that information are left unspoken, deliberately fudged, or denied outright. Of course patients and relatives do frequently feel the need to protect themselves from the pain of too much truth and, over the course of an illness, may move in and out of periods of denial. However, it is important to remember that denial is the prerogative of the patient, not of the staff. In lectures, palliative care nurses frequently tell me that they do not consider themselves to have the right to impart information. Nurses find their own ways of dealing with this dilemma. Some insist it is their right, their duty. Some work hard at the role of patient advocate, building bridges between doctor and patient when it is necessary. In rare situations teamwork amongst all professions is so well developed that the task of communication is freely shared. But too often nurses feel required to hedge and avoid patients' questions about the progress of the illness or about the implications of any information. In these situations nurses invariably feel compromised. In his book *Helplessness and Hope*, Bruce Rumbold (1986:59) has this to say about hope:

> In actual clinical practice two operational ideas about hope can be distinguished. The first of these is that hope is something which patients retain as long as sufficient information is withheld from them ('Nothing should be said to take away the patient's hope'). The second, usually a fall-back position introduced when patients have inferred or been told their prognoses, is that hope is a belief system which can be delivered in propositional form (preferably by a chaplain).

I believe that both these pragmatic views of hope are quite inadequate; indeed that they are a travesty of real hope, hopelessness masquerading as hope. Hope is not the same thing as wishful thinking or unfounded optimism, nor is it merely a set of concepts to be given intellectual assent. Rather, hope has its birth in a realistic assessment of our situation, and is grounded in our experiences and the values by which we live.

I want to suggest that we need to find the courage to be more truthful before the death, long before all treatment options are exhausted, before even the regime of treatment is considered and launched. We need to examine our desire to protect patients and families from the truth of cancer, our desire to protect them by withholding information, our desire to protect them by doing yet more tests, our desire to find one more aggressive treatment option, our desire to project the failures of treatment onto ourselves or, worse still, onto the patients. (In ward meetings I have often heard baldly stated: 'She failed her chemotherapy'.) I want to suggest we ask ourselves who it is we are protecting. We need to remind ourselves of the fact of our own humanity and to acknowledge our own limitations. We need to redefine our model of successful care so that a failure in treatment does not have to mean that we have failed.

Faced with a cancer diagnosis and with a truthful presentation of treatment options and prognosis, it is normal and healthy for patients to go through a period of introspection and soul-searching, very often accompanied by depression — what has come to be called anticipatory grief, a grief that looks ahead to the possibility of death. This depression brings with it the so-called negative feelings: sorrow, resentment, anger and rage, envy, regret, and even shame. To be around anyone experiencing such grief is always uncomfortable. But it should not be viewed with alarm, nor even as an unfortunate aberration in the 'desirable' pattern of the upwardly emotionally mobile fighting spirit. As in normal healthy grieving over the death of a loved relative or friend, this depression is an absolutely necessary part of the process of facing the possibility or the fact of loss — loss of part of one's body, loss of a hope in a particular outcome, loss of one's whole identity, loss of a future, loss of a secure world view that says such a thing cannot happen to me, loss of life itself. But it is not only anticipatory grief. It is present grief because these losses are experienced as little deaths, here and now, deaths that demand to be grieved. We need not fear such depression if we can learn to recognise these moments as little deaths that need to be grieved, if we can become more familiar with the pattern of grieving and with the truth that good grief can uncover the tender resilience that is real hope. In fact, once we recognise this pattern in the responses of patients, we begin to recognise it everywhere — even in ourselves, in our own responses to our work as well as in our personal lives. (Nurses may uncover old emotional wounds in themselves which had been forgotten or neglected. When this happens, nurses are in a good position to seek out professional help for themselves. Far from being a cause for shame, this is a mark of mature responsibility.)

The more familiar the pattern becomes, the less frightening it will appear and then the barriers we have so carefully constructed to protect ourselves will start to come down. When this happens it becomes gradually easier and easier to recognise the need to grieve our own little and big deaths. We will see how often we are tempted to offer less than the truth of ourselves in our dealings with one another. Recognising these moments in ourselves brings a growing awareness to our work. And awareness makes responsible choices possible. In his book *The Road Less Travelled*, psychiatrist Scott Peck (1978) has some helpful pointers to consider whenever we are confronted with the temptation to withhold truth:

1. Never speak falsehood.
2. Bear in mind that the act of withholding truth is always potentially a lie.
3. The decision to withhold truth should never be based on personal needs: for example, our need for power, need to be liked, a need to protect ourselves from challenge.
4. Conversely, the decision to withhold truth must always be based entirely on the needs of the person or people from whom the truth is being withheld.
5. The assessment of another's needs is an act of responsibility so complex that it can only be executed wisely when one operates out of genuine love/respect for the other.
6. The primary factor in the assessment of another's needs is the assessment of that person's ability to utilise the truth for their own spiritual growth. And we tend generally to underestimate this capacity.
NB The energy required for the self-discipline of honesty is far less than the energy required for secretiveness.

The story of Gina springs to mind: a young Italian woman, newly married, loved by the staff for her tough cheerfulness and frank open manner. Gina's melanoma initially responded to a combined regime of chemotherapy and radiotherapy. But as the year wore on, her health deteriorated, her pain became hard to manage and she needed to come in more and more frequently for radiotherapy. The staff then referred her to me, the pastoral counsellor. But it was clear Gina did not wish to talk with me. She was offended that her oncologist and the staff had 'pushed her off' onto me. I spoke with her oncologist and asked about Gina's prognosis. He said he was at his wits' end, that there was no more that he could do. 'She keeps asking me, "And after this, what next?"' I asked him how he answered her. 'I tell her we have always got something up our sleeves. But in truth, Linda, I haven't.' I said to him, 'I think Gina has guessed this for herself. She needs to hear that even when the last treatment is given and she is at the end of the road, you won't abandon her. She knows and trusts you and the nursing staff. She needs to hear this from you, not me. How else can she find the strength to die honestly, the way she has lived?'

Since after a patient dies there is no real choice for those left behind but to deal with the hard fact of death, and since we see that human nature is stronger than we generally believe, and since for all our medical and nursing technology and care we are not able to banish death from the scene, perhaps we need to examine with more courage our fear of the powerlessness we feel when there is no more we can do to save a life.

I am concerned here not only with what such denial of the reality of death does to patients and their relatives. I am concerned for what it does ultimately and here and now to ourselves and to one another in our work. It seems to me that for all their professional distance (a distance that at times is right and proper) nurses know in their bones that, at bottom, the line between patient and nurse is no line at all; that we, like them, are not immune from the ambivalence of our own human existence. I would even venture to suggest that, alongside the desire for excellence in nursing, be it in research or treatment or patient care, one of the unconscious reasons for working in the field is to struggle with this fact, to struggle with our own power and our own helplessness. This has always been a difficult thing to face, as the story about one of the original pioneers of cancer research in these lines from a poem called 'Power', by Adrienne Rich (1973), suggests:

> Today I was reading about Marie Curie:
> she must have known she suffered   from radiation sickness
> her body bombarded for years   by the element
> she had purified
> It seems she denied to the end
> the source of the cataracts on her eyes
> the cracked and suppurating skin   of her finger-ends
> till she could no longer hold   a test-tube or a pencil
>
> She died   a famous woman   denying
> her wounds
> denying
> her wounds   came   from the same source as her power

All professions who see themselves as being part of the fight against cancer (or any other disease) are particularly prone to Marie Curie's kind of denial. There are two realities to be faced here. First, fighting battles requires single-mindedness and sharp focus to be effective. Secondly, harmful side-effects are an inevitable part of frontier medicine, whether the risk is to the researcher, the pharmacist, the technician, the nurse or the patient. The power to heal seems always to lie uncomfortably close to the power to wound. The actual physical risks may be great or small. However, there are also other less tangible risks. When the roles of medicine and nursing are understood in terms of a fight against disease, the scene is set for winners and losers, success and failure, for the language of absolutes, of polarities, and the split between the two. We feel compelled to cling to whatever makes us feel powerful. We tend to reject whatever reminds us of our lack of power. Like Marie Curie, we deny our own wounds, afraid that if they are acknowledged they will rob us of our power.

If nurses could learn to see themselves as wounded healers, if we could acknowledge that each of us is always potentially patient as well as nurse, then we may well discover that in our shared humanity and mortality there is a power of a different order — a power that comes from the same source as our wounds. This kind of power is not easy to explain. It is known by experience, glimpsed fleetingly, uncovered in surprising and ordinary places, when least expected. It is hard to speak about it without betraying it. And yet, when we touch this power, we know. In the midst of a moment of vulnerable powerlessness, offering care without hope of cure, laid low by our fragility, yet daring to accept that we are not in control, we are surprised to find ourselves more deeply connected within ourselves and to one another. We discover that our wounds and our power belong together. And this discovery brings a lively hope, even in the face of death. This is my understanding of spirituality. Nurses do not have to be religious to grasp this spiritual potential. In fact, those who call themselves religious have sometimes not grasped it at all.

Religious people and sceptics alike are often so afraid of experiences that may not fit their particular frames of reference that they stop noticing and wondering altogether. In the words of the German philosopher, Rilke:

> That is at bottom the only courage that is demanded of us: to have courage for the most strange, the most singular and the most inexplicable that we may encounter. That mankind has in this sense been cowardly has done life endless harm; the experiences that are called 'visions', the whole so-called 'spirit-world', death, all those things that are so closely akin to us, have by daily parrying been so crowded out by life that the senses with which we could have grasped them are atrophied. To say nothing of God. (As quoted in Matthiesson, 1978)

The discovery that our power truly does come from the same source as our wounds helps us to see the nurse as wounded healer, to see the patient in every nurse, . . . and the nurse in every patient. To explore this mystery is to open ourselves to the realm of spirituality; to the gifts of wonder, heightened awareness, deeper connections, and the poss-ibilities of a fuller life even in the face of suffering and death.

REFERENCES

Matthiesson P (1989): *The Snow Leopard*. London: HarperCollins.

Peck MS (1978): *The Road Less Travelled* — a new psychology of love, traditional values and spiritual growth. Melbourne: Rider.

Rich A (1984): *The Fact of a Doorframe:* Poems Selected and New, 1950–1984. New York and London: WW Norton & Company, Inc.

Rumbold B (1986): *Helplessness and Hope* — pastoral care in terminal illness. London: SCM Press.

Worden JW (1983): *Grief Counselling and Grief Therapy*. London: Tavistock Publications.

OTHER READING

Nouwen HJM (1972): *The Wounded Healer* — ministry in contemporary society. New York: Doubleday and Co. Inc.

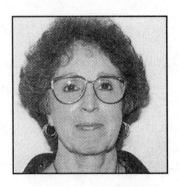

JACQUELINE KINSEY BAMBERY
RN, RM, BN, DipTh, AIMM

Jacquie Bambery is a registered nurse and midwife with a post-registration Bachelor of Nursing from Deakin University in Geelong, Australia. At the time this chapter was written, she was in her last semester of a Bachelor of Education at La Trobe University in Melbourne and was also undertaking a Diploma of Freelance Journalism through the Australian College of Journalism in Sydney. The holder of a Diploma of Theology, she claims no religious affiliation but has a long-standing interest in the spirituality of all people and finds the teaching of Tibetan Buddhism dynamic and relevant.

Jacquie's background is diverse and includes a number of years on the Spinal Injuries Unit at Austin Hospital in Melbourne where she also set up the first School of Post-Basic Nursing Education. She has both teaching and management experience and is a member of the Australian Institute of Management. Jacquie has also worked in Northern India, running a mobile tuberculosis clinic in the Himalayan foothills. She is currently in private practice which includes community-based pastoral care and a counselling service. She is writing a book, which she hopes will be accepted for publication, about grief and bereavement being a community experience and therefore a community responsibility.

Chapter 4

SPIRITUALITY
AS A HEALING FORCE

INTRODUCTION

Spirituality is a complex phenomenon, the definition of
which has occupied the minds of thinkers throughout the
centuries. In a recent radio interview the interviewer asked a
young Australian doctor currently working in Somalia
whether or not many aid workers choose to work in war-
torn countries for spiritual reasons. The doctor replied,
'Well, I guess some do go for religious reasons.' The doctor
is not alone in assuming that spirituality and religion are
synonymous. I suggest, however, that they are not.

In most of the literature I have read over many years
concerning what is termed 'the spiritual needs' of clients,
this area of client care is seen primarily as the domain of
pastoral carers. Pastoral care as we know it in Australia and
other Western cultures has its history within the ministry of
the Christian church (although people of all religious
persuasions are equally cared for). The pastoral carers who
work in our hospitals are an essential component of the
care team.

However, my concern lies in the trend that exists for some nurses to confuse the religious with the spiritual. In so doing I am convinced that, in many instances, our clients and the significant others in their lives are not holistically cared for and nurtured by the nurse.

What I offer you in this chapter are ideas, not opinions fixed like concrete in my mind, but a glimpse into my ongoing and ever-evolving view of spirituality — what it is and what it implies within the uniqueness of the nurse–client relationship.

ATTEMPTING A DEFINITION OF SPIRIT AND SPIRITUALITY

Smith (1988) in his book *The Concept of the Spiritual* writes almost 400 pages in discussing the definitions and concept of spirituality. I, however, have selected four words — psyche, soul, spirit and mind — as being the most commonly used when attempts are made to describe humans as being more than their material body. The Greek word for both soul and mind is Psyche, the root of English words such as psychology, psychiatry and psychosomatic. *The Concise Oxford Dictionary of Current English* edited by Fowler and Fowler in 1964 says that both the Greek 'pneuma' and the Latin 'spiritus', for breath (Fowler and Fowler 1964:936, 1236) are synonymous with 'anima', the Latin for soul (Glanz, Anderson and Anderson, 1990:67) from which is derived the word 'animate', translated as 'to breathe life into' (Fowler and Fowler, 1964:45). Here, therefore, is a sense that the spirit or soul is that which makes living things alive. Hegler, a German philosopher, used the word 'Geist', which translates as both spirit and mind, to suggest spirit is an I, different from matter (Flew, 1984:139). Sometimes, when we are endeavouring to define who we are as distinct from someone else, we might use a phrases such as 'Me, the person I am inside myself'. Plato and Socrates (Flew, 1984:331) identified the soul with the person who reasons, decides and acts. They assumed that this person of soul is 'not the familiar creature of flesh and blood but rather is the incorporeal [not composed of matter] occupant and even prisoner in and director of the corporeal [material] being'. Spirituality, therefore, could be summarised as the nonmaterial dimension of each human being, that which gives each and all its life.

To describe people, therefore, as 'more' or 'less' spiritual than others is erroneous. Perhaps what we observe in someone described as 'very spiritual' is what both Rogers and Maslow refer to as the human's tendency for self-actualisation.

> Maslow loosely defined self-actualisation as 'the full use and exploitation of talents, capacities, potentialities etc' . . . Self-actualisation is not a static state. It is an ongoing process in which one's capacities are fully, creatively and joyfully utilised (Fadiman and Frager, 1994:471).

Rogers speaks of this self-actualising tendency as an urge that:

> . . . is part of the process of all living things. It is the urge to expand, extend, develop, mature — the tendency to express and activate all the capacities to the extent that such activation enhances the . . . self (cited in Fadiman and Frager, 1994:471).

Obviously a person moving progressively towards self-actualisation, developing the wellspring of their potential as a unique individual I, would demonstrate a level of maturity and many characteristics (love, generosity, patience etc.) that would attract notice and praise. It is because self-actualisation is achieved gradually that we hear people voice erroneous interpretations of degrees of spirituality.

Frank Lopez is a member of the Marist Fathers' Province in Australia and Director of the Marist Centre for Pastoral Care Distance Education Programs in Hunter's Hill, New South Wales. He demonstrates a forward-thinking capacity to deal with the issue of pastoral care within the context of today's society with its increasing religious pluralism (many religions) and secularisation ('when religion ceases to permeate or dominate society as a whole') (Lopez, 1994:131). Whilst Lopez's writings reveal the depth of his religious life and personal relationship with God, he nevertheless affirms that spirituality and religion are not synonymous, that spirituality existed before religion, indwelling our human status.

> Spirituality is . . . a human reality . . . it focuses on the human spirit of both believers and 'non-believers' and on their lives as a whole . . . spirituality may or may not include God . . . may or may not be explicitly religious or Church-related . . . (Lopez, 1994:128-129).

Thus, spirituality exists as a dimension of the humanness of each human being and is separate from and not to be confused with religion, but is not in opposition to religion and may involve a person's religious beliefs where these exist.

SPIRITUALITY IN CONCERT — THE SHARING OF HUMANNESS IN THE NURSE–CLIENT RELATIONSHIP

> When you work you are a flute through whose heart the whispering of the hours turns to music . . . Work is love made visible. And if you cannot work with love but only with distaste, it is better that you should leave your work and sit at the gate of the temple and take alms of those who work with joy (Gibran, 1970:32 and 35).

Having looked at spirituality as the life force which indwells all human beings, the inference I make is that when nurses speak of the spiritual needs of clients they are in fact referring to the total needs of the whole human/spirit person and not to religious needs which may or may not exist. Where clients have needs of a religious nature it is appropriate to involve a pastoral worker in assisting the client with exploring these. However, in the day-to-day life of client and nurse, what exists is a unique, individual or personal I that is the nurse in relationship with a unique, individual I that is the client. This relationship is, for both of them, a lived experience. It concerns the human existence of both in union with each other. Heidegger, a German philosopher, describes being-in-the-world in terms of 'enjoining oneself' or 'being accessible to'. The German words used are translated as 'presencing oneself' (Benner and Wrubel, 1989:13).

> This ability to presence oneself; to be with a patient in a way that acknowledges your shared humanity, is the base of much of nursing as a caring practice . . . To presence oneself with another means that you are available to understand and be with someone. Presencing oneself contrasts with standing aloof and outside the situation . . .

This 'shared humanity' or sharing of humanness is an activity of human life in which the spirit dimension, the I of each, connects or unites. This, I suggest, is spirituality — the sharing of humanness one to another. The title of this book, *Spirituality: The Heart of Nursing*, thus becomes *The Sharing of Humanness: The Heart of Nursing*. This sharing of humanness describes how we are in the world. Heidegger described 'man's mode of being in the world' using 'Dasein' which translates into 'being there'.

> . . . being-in-the-world is characterised by relatedness to surrounding objects and members of his community, in terms of being concerned with and caring about them (Flew, 1984:83).

65

SPIRITUALITY, THE SHARING OF HUMANNESS AS A HEALING FORCE

Nurse as ordinary person — nurse's perspective

Professor Bev Taylor, who is the Foundation Chair in Nursing at the Southern Cross University in northern New South Wales, is extraordinarily gifted in describing the richness of people's lived experience and has published a wealth of literature on the subject. At a national nursing conference held in Melbourne in 1991 she presented a paper entitled 'The dialectic of the nurse as person: ordinary nurses perceived as extraordinarily effective'. The paper explores nurse as person and Taylor suggests that:

> . . . we tend to categorise people into discrete compartments that are convenient for us, but nevertheless have a tendency to limit people's essential humanness — in order to make our worlds predictable and manageable, we tend to draw sharp distinctions between nurses and patients, unwittingly robbing all or some of their inherent richness as unique entities (Taylor, 1991:9).

Taylor further suggests that the concept of person changes its meaning 'if we as humans are encouraged to see people in terms of their oneness rather than by their separateness' (Taylor, 1991:9). She proceeds to explore the nature of the ordinariness of both patient and nurse, emphasising a 'relationship of reciprocity rather than a unilateral dispensation of professional help' (Taylor, 1991:14). Taylor questions whether, in the process of 'becoming sophisticated in nursing skills and knowledge, nurses may have lost sight of their essential nature as people' (Taylor, 1991:14).

This nature of ordinariness that Taylor discusses, of both client and nurse, and the sharing of it in a reciprocal relationship, I view as an antecedent to the concept of spirituality as the sharing of humanness. Within the merging of the ordinariness and the extraordinariness (the unique personal I that they each are) of both nurse and client, the opportunity exists for healing to take place toward a state of health. But what counts as healing, who is healed and what is implied in the term health?

The West Germanic word for health is 'hailia' translated as 'whole' and the Germanic 'hailaz', for heal, is translated as 'whole', implying a connection between the two (Fowler and Fowler, 1964:565). In nursing, the concept of holistic care generates from the contention that a person is not '. . . a composite of a variety of subsystems such as physiological, psychological, social and so forth' (Leddy and Pepper, 1989:211). Reducing people to component parts '. . . destroys or distorts the integrity [wholeness, soundness] of the whole' (Flynn, 1980:9, cited in Leddy and Pepper, 1989). How we as nurses seek to prevent the health or wholeness (soundness) of our clients being compromised is through employment of the caring practice of our individual and collective skills. Both the aim and the outcome of this practice ought to be healing, which is a continuous process.

> Healing isn't something you do and put away on a shelf . . . It's a dynamic equilibrium that has to be maintained daily (Barasch, 1995:371).

Thus, in each separate, mutually shared episode involving nurse and client, there is a movement forward which I believe is an occasion for joy. This is nurse (as ordinary person) and client sharing their human/spirit selves in a relationship which, I believe, is a healing force. Both nurse and client carry within themselves the wounds and scars that life inevitably exposes all of us to. The nurse takes on the role, therefore, of wounded healer, yet my experience has been that, in the act of applying measures geared toward aiding my client's healing process, I have walked away from the bedside feeling infused with energy despite my tiredness and sadness at my client's illness. The aim of caring and nurturing is healing, and just as the relationship is one of mutuality, so too, I suggest, is the outcome of the healing that takes place.

We commence our lives dependent and move in the growth process to become independent in young adulthood and take personal responsibility for ourselves. However, in sharing humanness, the focus moves to include others in an interdependent way where we 'operate in terms of mutual understanding, co-operation, valuing difference and demonstrating a capacity to care' (Lopez, 1994:67). This is something of how I perceive spirituality.

Nurse as ordinary person — client perspective

Tony Moore is currently Medical Director of Hampton Rehabilitation Hospital in Melbourne. Prior to this appointment, whilst he was driving to work one day, his car was hit by a 30-tonne semitrailer, leaving both him and his car crushed. In his book *Cry of the Damaged Man* (Moore, 1991) he speaks with great skill and honesty about the best and worst of being a patient and about 'the depths of his despair and profound isolation'. Below is an account of how one nurse's sharing of humanness helped him:

Someone who did help . . . in the early days was one of the
evening nurses. She came in each night at about half past eleven
. . . even though she was off duty at eleven . . . and if I knew
I couldn't sleep . . . she would come in to talk . . . Nothing
upset her. Everything was taken with natural acceptance . . .
She was unpretentious, unaffected and one of God's children
. . . She had an infallible instinct for human suffering . . . She
never pushed or probed. 'I only come in here to drink your
Baileys,' she said one night after I told her she was a good-
hearted soul . . . When I left the ward I gave her a book. 'Jesus,'
she said, 'I was hoping for a bottle of Baileys' (Moore,
1991:34-35).

Nurse as ordinary person — a relative's perspective

We have taken a few pages to reflect upon the sharing of
humanness (spirituality) as the essence of nursing and have
centred our attention primarily upon this sharing as it occurs
between nurse and client. However, a holistic approach to
nursing is inclusive of the significant others in the client's life.
Scherper-Hughes and Locke (1987) point out that 'Sickness
is not just an isolated event, nor an unfortunate brush with
nature. It is a form of communication . . . ' (cited in Benner
and Wrubel, 1989:9–10) which becomes part of the lived
experience of both the client and those with whom they share
their life. This sickness, this vehicle of communication,
disrupts the meanings and understanding that people have
and therefore changes the way the world is viewed.

Further dislocation of meaning can occur, for example, if
the client and loved ones are informed that the sickness is
terminal. Subsequent events which occur and which are

perceived as negative further impact upon and distort the meaning and understanding of reality as it is perceived to exist for that person. The adage that 'what is real for one is not necessarily real for another', is true.

> The personal quality of meanings and the importance they have in the private worlds of individuals are of tremendous significance to workers in helping professions. The moment we understand other people in terms of personal meaning, a great deal that was formerly puzzling or inexplicable becomes meaningful and reasonable (Combs and Gonzalez, 1994:71-72).

This lived experience of sickness communicates itself in pain and suffering, in lost dreams and shattered hopes and in grief. It alienates and isolates and within this isolation the one affected focuses totally on the pain of the immediate situation, often with feelings of hopelessness. Both the client and the client's loved ones can enter into this alien place of isolation. Into this arena walks the nurse, by choice, to share the ordinariness of being human and the extraordinariness of being a unique spiritual I.

Whether or not this sharing of humanness or spirituality is experienced as a healing force is dependent upon the nature of the relationship the nurse initiates. Martin Buber, a Jewish philosopher and theologian, makes a radical distinction between two basic attitudes of which people are capable, described as I–Thou and I–It. I–Thou designates a relation between subject and subject, a relation of reciprocity and mutuality. I–It is the relation between subject and object, involving some form of utilisation or control, the object being wholly passive. The I in the two situations also differs. In the I–Thou it appears only in the context of the relationship and cannot be involved independently, whereas in the I–It situation the I is an observer and only partly involved (Flew, 1984:50). The I–Thou relationship is akin to the act of 'presencing oneself' spoken of earlier in this chapter, where the nurse 'stands alongside and not aloof looking on'. In forestry the word 'nurse' is used to denote a tree planted as shelter to others (Fowler and Fowler, 1964:827).

Such a capacity to bond and share with, to become one with, requires constancy of purpose and compassion.

> What is compassion? It is not simply a sense of sympathy or caring for the person suffering, not simply a warmth of heart toward the person before you, or a sharp clarity of recognition of their needs and pain, it is also a sustained and practical determination to do whatever is possible and necessary to help alleviate their suffering (Soygal Rinpoche, 1995:4 June).

This 'sustained and practical determination' that Soygal Rinpoche speaks of as being necessary in order to do 'whatever is possible and necessary to help alleviate suffering', must have a power source. I believe that power is love which results in caring. Maslow includes love needs and a sense of belonging in his list of basic psychological needs. 'All people have belonging and love needs' (Fadiman and Frager, 1994:469). Do nurses remember this in times of caring for clients with a protracted illness where repeated hospitalisations separate husband from wife, child from parent? There is, I believe, an aspect of surrogacy in the nurse's role at such times.

Does this spirit energy, love which results in caring, exist as an aspect of the humanness of each and every nurse? I believe that the potential to give and receive love indwells all of us, but that we make a choice regarding how far we develop our individual potentiality. Nurses, however, are human beings

71

with their own needs, hopes, fears, dreams and problems, just like the clients and their family members. Each is at a varying stage of personal growth. I became acutely aware of this when my husband was dying three years ago. What follows is an extract from my personal journal.

I always remember when I worked in clinical bedside nursing that it was commonly stated by the nursing staff that doctors and nurses or members of their families made the worst patients and relatives. There was often at such times a discernible expectancy that 'somewhere along the line' there would be problems. I was conscious of keeping this in mind when Ron became ill and consequently I felt awkward about approaching the nurses with questions and certainly avoided any hint of criticism or comment that might be interpreted as dissatisfaction.

The ward was always busy and the nurses worked hard. They were generally 'a good bunch'. However, the news of Ron's misdiagnosis and the enormity of its implications swept over me like a tidal wave and as he entered the last two horrifying months of his life I could barely sustain my inner strength. I felt that emotionally I was unravelling and disintegrating. I was conscious of a void filled only with pain and terror. I entered an alien and foreign place.

The Pastoral Care worker sometimes visited when I was there. She was a volunteer and liked to say 'Hello' but if I tried to say how I really felt she became obviously uncomfortable, looked at her watch and said she'd have to go.

The nurses were 'there' for Ron — I can't complain about his care — but always I perceived that I was seen as a nurse and it's as if they expected that to somehow influence my experience of being a grieving wife. It was a case of 'the nurse whose husband's our patient' rather than 'the wife of a man who's dying'.

Towards the end I watched in horror Ron's suffering and I became someone else — someone I didn't know — and I can't explain that. Two days before he died I became agitated — I think when I look back that's what I'd call it. Ron was restless, in pain and choking to death bit by bit. The doctor said afterwards he hadn't thought that he would die then. I think I knew, but somehow the notion hadn't surfaced into conscious awareness.

One day a group of nurses came to turn Ron. I'd always been permitted to be involved in his care. They were good about that. They were having difficulty lifting him and I made a suggestion — that's all I was doing — but one of the nurses, in front of the rest of the staff, told me off and accused me of speaking rudely to one of her colleagues.

I was startled and remarked, 'I wasn't being rude', but this evoked further rebuke so I turned and stared out of the window. I felt a sense of not belonging and not being cared about. I became the nurse who was the difficult relative. They left the room except for the nurse to whom I had supposedly been rude. I remember thinking 'I haven't got the strength for this' and I braced myself for what might now be said. She crossed the room as I protested that I hadn't meant to be rude. She said, 'I know,' as she held me in a firm hug which said, 'I care, I understand and I'm here.' Our tears flowed, wetting both our shoulders.

That was one of only three or four occasions in sixteen months in which I felt as if anyone really understood what was happening to me. It was the only acknowledgment that my husband was dying.

Taylor uses the term 'intuneness' to describe an aspect of ordinariness 'within which we are sensitive to our feelings and express them as a legitimate part of ourselves' (Taylor, 1991:13).

> In nursing, intuneness creates the potential for patients and nurses to acknowledge and express the polarity of their feelings . . . clearing away the debris of rationality to face up to and embrace the rawness of emotions which, expressed, unblock the streams of human reactivity and cause our life energies to flow a little easier. Intuneness knows the other with whom it seeks to share its feelings, because it knows its own feeling nature as part of itself (Taylor, 1991:13).

Is caring an essential component of shared humanness? Neville (1989:18) asserts that 'the . . . spirit perspective looks for the non-obvious, the invisible, the poem hidden in the hard reality'. This is caring!

Is Sharing Humanness the Heart of Nursing?

Sharing humanness is spirituality in action, requiring sustained and practical determination to do whatever is possible to alleviate suffering. This is Soygal Rinpoche's 'compassion'. What the sustaining and empowering ingredient of compassion is, is love, symbolised in the myth of Psyche, a beautiful young woman whom the ancient Greeks recognised in the butterfly and whom medieval writers saw as an image of the soul in search of God (Neville, 1989:3).

Eros (Cupid) was love, the force responsible for all creation (if present) and responsible for destruction (if absent). It's a story of how the soul (Psyche) is drawn by love (Eros) through a slow, painful, shadowy initiation and transformed into a new way of 'being'. Thus Eros marries Psyche and she becomes immortal (Neville, 1989:3). Psyche and Eros, the personal I ensouled in love, is the transformative healing force of the sharing of humanness. This is the heart of nursing.

REFERENCES

Barasch MI (1995): *The Healing Path, A Soul Approach to Illness*. New York: Penguin.

Benner P and Wrubel J (1989): *The Primacy of Caring Stress and Coping in Health and Illness*. California: Addison-Wesley.

Combs AW and Gonzales DM (1994): *Helping Relationships: Basic Concepts for the Helping Professions*. Massachusetts: Allyn and Bacon.

Fadiman J and Frager R (1994): *Personality and Personal Growth*. New York: Harper Collins College Publishers.

Flew A (1984): *A Dictionary of Philosophy*. London: Pan Books Ltd.

Fowler HW and Fowler FG (eds) (1964): *The Concise Oxford Dictionary of Current English*. London: Oxford University Press.

Gibran K (1970): *The Prophet*. London: Heinemann.

Glanz WD, Anderson KN, Anderson LE (eds) (1990): *Mosby's Medical, Nursing and Allied Health Dictionary* (3rd edn). St Louis: The CV Mosby Company.

Leddy S and Pepper JM (1989): *Conceptual Bases of Professional Nursing*. Philadelphia: JB Lippincott Company.

Lopez F (1994): *Pastoral Care in an Emerging World*. Hunter's Hill, NSW, Australia: Marist Centre for Pastoral Care, Department of Distance Learning.

Moore T (1991): *Cry of the Damaged Man*. Sydney: Picador.

Neville B (1989): *Educating Psyche*. Melbourne: Collins Dove.

Rinpoche Soygal (1995): *Glimpse after Glimpse: Daily Reflections on Living and Dying*. London: Rider.

Smith SG (1988): *The Concept of the Spiritual: An Essay in First Philosophy*. Philadelphia: Temple Press.

Taylor B (1991): The dialectic of the nurse as patient: ordinary nurses perceived as extraordinarily effective. In: *Science Reflectivity and Nursing Care: Exploring the Dialectic,* Proceedings of the National Nursing Conference, pp. 9-14. Melbourne: Quality Health Forums Pty Ltd.

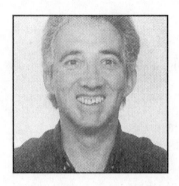

TONY BUSH
RN, RPN, DipAppSc, BAppSc, MPHC

After Tony Bush had worked in a number of Australian States and overseas countries in numerous clinical roles, it became apparent to him that spirituality is common to all people, regardless of their background. In recent years, since completing postgraduate studies in palliative care, Tony has found it possible to develop a model of spiritual care for use not only in a clinical capacity but also in his personal life. This appreciation of existential aspects has reaffirmed his belief that spiritual care really does have a place in nursing curricula and that an exploration of such matters will encourage a student to undertake a personal journey of reflection not just as a nurse, but also as a person. At present Tony coordinates a postgraduate course in palliative care in which students are introduced to the topic of spirituality. This is a very popular aspect of the course which has led Tony to investigate some educational matters involved in facilitating the exploration of such a seemingly nebulous subject.

Chapter 5

SPIRITUALITY IN CARE

A current nursing focus is on the practice of holistic nursing and all that it entails. According to Burkhardt (1989), holistic care includes the domain of spirit and spirituality, and Ross (1995) and Buckle (1993) say that spirituality is a cornerstone of holism and accordingly has a role to play in the delivery of nursing care.

While many nurses say they are very familiar with holistic nursing, the nursing care they carry out concentrates on the various biopsychosocial needs of their patients. The average nurse is apparently not as able to meet their patients' spiritual needs, even though these are a feature of holism (Narayanasamy, 1993). Many nurses avoid spiritual matters in their patient care, as they believe them to be outside their job description or beyond their ability (Narayanasamy, 1993). Yet in order to promote patients' health, well-being and quality of life, it has been suggested that nurses ought to appreciate that if spiritual care is not being provided, could it be said of nurses that they are not doing that which they are prepared for — to provide care?

Caring in nursing incorporates empathy, sensitivity and compassion and these are all qualities with which nurses are familiar (Diers, 1990). These same qualities are described by Price, Stevens and LaBarre (1995) as being very useful in the promotion of spiritual well-being, so nurses are probably not so unfamiliar with practices relating to spiritual care as they might think.

Narayanasamy (1993) suggests that, in patient care, nurses avoid matters of a spiritual nature as they believe them to be outside their clinical domain; this perception of what is meant by spirituality overlooks the fact that nurses also have spiritual needs, that such needs are not peculiar to patients.

Does this mean then that nurses are somehow different from other people? For many nurses this perception may ring true, as they were inducted into a way of thinking by their educators and hospital colleagues which discouraged 'getting involved' with patients. As a result some nurses do not allow their own contextual background to enrich their contacts with patients. They have evolved into nurses who happen to be people rather than people who happen to be nurses.

Yet every person is a spiritual being with a spiritual dimension and so nurses themselves have spiritual needs which can be used as a basis for a beginning spiritual exploration between patients and themselves. Unfortunately, this exchange is infrequently undertaken, as spiritual care is often interpreted by carers to mean religious care, and therefore comes under the domain of formally prepared religious persons, such as ministers, rabbis, or priests. Such confusion between the terms 'spiritual care' and 'religious care' is common and it is not surprising that nurses may be perplexed given the multitude of definitions of the term spirituality.

SPIRITUALITY DESCRIBED

Whilst the concept of spirituality is often associated with religion there is a difference between these terms. 'Spiritual' can be described as 'pertaining to the spirit of Man' and 'spirit' as the 'breath of life which gives life to the physical organism' (Stoter, 1995:3).

A further examination of these descriptions indicates that the spiritual dimension facilitates a search for meaning in life and for meaning related to concerns and commitments. How often must nurses witness sick and vulnerable patients attempting to make sense of such seemingly nebulous concerns? Indeed, how often must nurses try to make sense of their own spiritual concerns when trying to find some meaning in an apparently meaningless situation, such as caring for an incurably ill child?

Although there are many definitions of the spiritual dimension, an early definition by Renetzky (1979) appears to include all the facets that have been mentioned so far:

- the need to find meaning, purpose and fulfilment in life, suffering and death;
- the need for hope/will to live; and
- the need for belief and faith in self, others and God.

These components are formed and influenced by a person's life experiences and so the expression of one's spiritual needs will reflect an individual's cultural, personal and professional background. In a contemporary Australian context the diversity of cultural and ethnic backgrounds also means a variety of spiritual expressions. It is common for nurses to witness these in their clinical practice, and for them to begin to recognise similarities and differences between spirituality and religiosity.

For many patients and nurses alike, spirituality and religion have the same meaning. These people often have a clear personal understanding of spiritual matters. Their search for meaning is encapsulated within their religion, which can be described as the formal framework of beliefs that assists in the practical expression of spirituality (Grey, 1994). Usually, such a religious structure has a number of rituals and practices, which many nurses are used to seeing associated with the presence of a clergyman, such as the administration of Holy Communion. But for others, who may not have such a prescriptive faith, their expression of spirituality may take place in other ways, such as through their relationships with significant others, their personal achievements in life or any other factors which have been given personal significance as a result of their upbringing and life experiences. As a means of adapting to or coping with illness the spiritual dimension takes on a considerable significance for patients, who often turn to the nurse as a means of expressing their spiritual needs (Harrison, 1993). It's fair to say that most people will keep private their innermost concerns and it is only in times of crisis, such as being hospitalised, that a patient may take time to reflect upon spirituality. This awakening of need may also act as a catalyst for the nurse to reflect upon their own life and so begin to discover their own priorities and values, thus commencing a search for spiritual meaning.

SEARCH FOR MEANING

The search for meaning is commonly associated with persons who have a terminal illness although there are indications that all areas of nursing will encounter patients who have commenced this journey. The need to find purpose and meaning in one's life is a universal trait, necessary for the maintenance of life; it's considered a feature of a well-developed personality and can prevent feelings of uselessness in old age (Ross, 1995). For many medical and surgical patients entering into a health care setting, there may arise a need to find meaning in their illness and subsequent removal from their own familiar environment (Harrington, 1995). Traditionally, such a conscious act of reflection does not usually commence for many people until they are faced with a potentially threatening illness or until they have reached a certain maturity, however that may be defined. For many youthful nurses preoccupied with their daily activities, such a journey of introspection may not occur until they are faced with their own crises. How much more rewarding it would be for nurses to have given consideration to this question before they are exposed to any threats to their integrity.

A number of nurses are able to find significant meaning in their work and consequently express feelings of fulfilment and self-worth. If this investment in life is considered so important to one's well-being, what of those people who are unable to find any meaning in life at all? For example, could the increasing incidence in youth suicide and the escalating numbers of people seeking counselling be due to spiritual distress resulting from living without meaning, culminating in feelings of emptiness and despair (Burnard, 1989)? Perhaps a contributing cause to this situation may be the increasing objectification of people by our contemporary society, which is alienating people from themselves (Fromm, 1974). Could it be that the reintegration of such persons with the world and the provision of a balance between the negative and positive aspects of their life take place only when people's spiritual needs are recognised by those who profess to care?

Often patients attempt to uncover a meaning in their life through reminiscing and ruminating about their past experiences; they try to find a connection from one aspect of their life to another. It is common to hear patients utter statements like 'I've wasted my life', or questions such as, 'Why me?', 'What use am I?', or 'What do my family really think of me?' (Price, Stevens and LaBarre, 1995; Doyle, 1992).

A helpful method of assisting with the search for meaning can be by asking the patient to describe their earliest memories of home and school and then proceeding through a description of their significant life recollections. Not all of these may appear relevant to the nurse; however, it is not the nurse who creates meaning for the patient, but rather the patient developing their own meaning in their own way. As already indicated, this may come about by linking events and people, past, present and future, and bringing them together in the patient's present moment (Fox, 1988). Such a search often leads to a re-evaluation of one's priorities, and the realisation that human life can rise above the present circumstances (Birch, 1990).

For the nurse who recognises a patient's search and assists in the process, the personal rewards are potentially enormous. The experience will provide an opportunity to reflect on the nurse's own values and priorities. It is a chance to start a personal journey of reflection which will help to uncover meaning both in professional and personal life.

Naturally there are no 'quick fix' answers to such a perplexing question as what is the purpose and meaning in life.

Such a question may arise when a patient is faced with a serious health threat, for example, someone awaiting the results of pathology tests, or for those facing the prospect of surgery. The nurse who wishes to accompany a patient along the path of self-discovery may assist more fully by appreciating the uniqueness of the patient's role as a person, and sharing with that person those life events which all people experience, such as relationships, successes, failures, wishes and aspirations. A nurse can remind the patient that they are valuable not because of their life's achievements, but simply because they exist (Fox, 1988). Through this acknowledgment and affirmation of the patient's worth, the nurse can create the circumstances necessary for the patient to create their own meaning.

NEED FOR HOPE

Hope is a feature of human existence and is regarded as an intrinsic element of life, providing a reason for living, a sense of well-being and a means of preventing the pain of despair (Ross, 1995; Carson, 1989). This is a very big claim indeed, and yet nurses regularly witness those patients who have lost hope seemingly give up the will to live, even when their illness may not be life threatening.

It appears that there is some evidence to support the notion that hope is fundamental to a person's survival and its loss can lead to premature death; if a person has no control over life events, then the effects of helplessness/hopelessness can result in death, akin to 'passive suicide' (Ross, 1993, 1995; Renetzky, 1979; Limandri and Boyle, 1978). The onset of hopelessness can be attributed partly to the illness, but any loss of control can arise from prolonged inactivity, isolation, a deteriorating physical state, a sense of abandonment, chronic stress and the onset of doubts about one's spiritual or religious beliefs (Urden, Davis and Thalan, 1992). On the other hand, nurses have also witnessed those seemingly 'hopeless' patients who recover from potentially fatal illnesses against all medical predictions. It appears there may be some basis to the popularly held belief that a will to live can give a person a better-than-even chance of overcoming a serious illness (Renetzky, 1979).

There does appear to be, however, a potential for health care professionals to unconsciously create helplessness in patients. Our contemporary society generally pays little attention to a person's spiritual growth and has replaced this domain with an emphasis on the tangible evidence of personal achievements, such as social status, work status or personal possessions. This has led to many people developing a reliance on themselves and their achievements. When a patient is in the care of another person, such beliefs are often very difficult to maintain, as there is now a reliance on other people who may or may not include the patient in any decision making relating to that patient's well-being. So much for the reliance on self.

Helplessness in nurses, and indeed doctors, is not uncommon, particularly in situations when it appears that these professionals are apparently unable to 'cure' someone. Some nurses may deal with their own helplessness by 'avoiding' the person. Whilst they may carry out essential tasks, there may be little of the personal interaction which nurses routinely employ. Most patients are sensitive to these situations and may interpret this as the nurses' reluctance to become involved with a 'hopeless case'. The patient may begin to perceive their situation as being hopeless and one which they are helpless to change. While this may be a time when the patient is in most need of hope, spiritual pain, alienation and despair can surface, as indicated by such phrases as, 'What's the point?', 'Leave me alone' (said either in anger or sadness) and 'Why bother?' (Fox, 1988; Rumbold, 1986). Since hope and the will to live are very similar, it would seem quite logical for any person perceived to be in a 'hopeless' situation to simply give up. A nurse is not required to offer false hopes to anyone, but rather to include the patient in clinical planning and decision making and to encourage the patient to actively use their own religious or spiritual beliefs as a means of maintaining hope. Victor Frankl, a survivor of the holocaust, recorded his experiences and reflections and concluded that, even in the presence of apparent hopelessness, he maintained hope by observing that a person is not lessened by suffering but by suffering without meaning (Frankl, 1964).

BELIEF IN SELF THROUGH LOVE

If we can assume that spirituality is a force that determines the well-being of a person and provides meaning and motivation in life, then how does this concept help us in our relationships with each other? Dare one suggest it is through love and compassion which provide the means for people to bond (Goodloe and Arreola, 1992)? Whilst this love can be experienced through human relationships, many people also seek it from God, using their own faith's practices. It has been argued by Fox (1988) that this love is a common link between all mankind and creates an awareness for us all that God is not apart from us but a part of us. But what if the patient does not have a formal belief in God? It does not appear to affect a patient adversely, though it appears that one's spiritual well-being is significantly more pronounced if one has a belief in God (Renetzky, 1979).

Many nurses have witnessed the sense of contentment which surrounds a very ill patient, following a visit from loved ones; but there are many patients in the health care system who do not have any formal religious beliefs, nor do they have any significant relationships with family and friends. This does not mean that their need for love is less, but rather they might seek acceptance and recognition of their personal worth from the nursing staff. It is all well and good to describe these concepts, but how can a nurse provide such care? One way has been described as taking the cues from the patient and 'being yourself . . . it comes through in your caring, in your loving, in your administrations' (Harrington, 1995:9). Is this enough though? Peck (1978) noted that the nurturing of a person's spiritual development requires components of care for self and the individual, a responsibility to provide care, a respect for self and the individual and sufficient knowledge to facilitate a person's search for acceptance.

Caregivers need to be able to recognise and respond to a patient's feelings, to be willing to enter into the person's experiences through the use of empathy and to respect that person's intrinsic worth. They should enjoy a patient's likeable personal qualities. They ought to acknowledge the various factors which can influence their own actions, such as feeling dispirited themselves. They should view new experiences, such as spirituality, not as an extra 'thing to do', but rather as an experience which offers an opportunity for personal reflection and development (Birch, 1990). Whilst this may appear straightforward enough, our society's objectification of people has diminished the capacity to love and to accept oneself as being worthy of love, although the need remains. It is not easy for a nurse to give unconditionally. One must be extremely comfortable with oneself and must also know when to stop or to hand over to someone with more expertise.

So far, it appears that the nurse is providing all the 'giving' and receiving little in return. Yet it is the nurturing of a person's spiritual development that creates the circumstances necessary for a nurse's own spiritual growth. Such sharing is described as love, and it is by the giving of unconditional love that the nurse is able to receive a reciprocated love from the patient (Peck, 1978). Most nurses can recall an occasion when a patient has given them a personal message of affection, gratitude and praise, and the comforting afterglow this created. Patients are not obliged to 'give of themselves' but usually do so, in response to nurses who, by 'giving of themselves', reaffirm that patient's worth; it is all done by promoting the patient's spiritual growth through love.

Undoubtedly there are some nurses who may deride this concept as being too 'soft' and not practical enough. But this aspect of caring has been described as being able to provide a mutual discovery of spirituality between patient and caregiver, and perhaps more importantly, to give meaning to one's own life. One lives the meaning of one's life (not 'simply having direction') when the focus of one's life is caring for others (Millison and Dudley, 1990; Mayerhoff, 1972). The benefits to a nurse are apparent, not just in a professional sense, but also in personal life.

As previously mentioned, a belief in God or a formalised religious belief may give a person a significant advantage in maintaining their spiritual well-being and subsequent quality of life. It appears that through this belief, a person has a belief in themselves and a sense of purpose (Ross, 1995). For many people, God is viewed as a God of love and so it is not surprising that many patients and nurses find a great satisfaction in being 'loved' (Fox, 1988). As people seek meaning and love from a spiritual being, so too they seek forgiveness in love from that same being. Some nurses can well recall patients for whom nothing seemed to work — treatments were ineffective, sleeping patterns were disrupted and they appeared genuinely unhappy. One such person was a middle-aged man admitted for a relatively minor procedure who appeared excessively fearful of the consequences of not waking up post-anaesthesia. As he professed a formal religious faith, a minister was asked to visit him and it transpired that he felt guilty about some previous transgression and needed to know he was forgiven. Following the minister's visit the man settled down quickly and expressed his relief at being reassured that his God was indeed a loving and forgiving God. Perhaps this is a gentle reminder for nurses that in the newfound excitement of being able to facilitate spiritual care, it is a wise nurse indeed who knows when to use the services of available clergy.

Providing Spiritual Care

The provision of spiritual care is seen by nurses and patients as being a legitimate area of practice (Harrington, 1995; Cella and Tross, 1986). Whilst it is relatively simple to understand the components of spirituality, it may be quite strange and disconcerting for nurses to actually facilitate a patient's exploration of spiritual needs. It is wise to remember that it is the patient who uncovers these needs not the nurse, so it may not be a case of a nurse 'doing something' for/to the patient, but rather 'being there' with the patient, whilst the discovery is taking place.

This 'being there' implies both a physical and a psychological presence and requires the development of trust between nurse and patient, respect for the patient's personal beliefs by all the nursing staff and, perhaps more importantly, the nurse being very aware of their own strengths and limitations (Clark and

Heidenreich, 1995; Stoter, 1995). It's probably true to say that most nurses have these qualities already and so may believe that when these are added to 'caring' it is enough to see the job through. Without wishing to dampen anyone's enthusiasm, it appears that the provision of spiritual support requires more than compassion; there is a need for the caregiver to be comfortable with spiritual matters, to have well-developed communication skills and to be prepared to become involved with a patient in all their dimensions (Rumbold, 1986). Good caring includes compassion and competence and when these two are combined it can transform despair into hope (Cassidy, 1988). Remember, though, to come to the patient without any prescriptive ideas of the 'right way' of facilitating spiritual care and be willing to share the context of the patient's life as they see it.

It seems that most nurses who practise spiritual care do so without being asked by the patient and often as a result of intuition. There is nothing wrong in a nurse feeling something is amiss in a patient and acting accordingly. If truth be known, it's probably true to say nurses base a lot of their interventions on clinical judgement, underpinned by the feeling that 'something is not quite right'. There are two areas that often give the clues — the nurse's use of eye contact and the patient's use of words.

Eye contact is a common feature of all patient–nurse encounters and is an invaluable aid to the development of a rapport based on respect. It can be described as, 'the first person-to-person touch from carer to patient' (Stoter, 1995:39). A nurse approaching a patient can ask silently, 'What do I really see — the equipment, the patient's physical appearance, their demeanour, or all of these things?' The follow-up silent question can be: 'What does the patient see in me — someone in a hurry, someone flustered and impatient or someone who has a genuine smile, an aura of calmness and an apparent willingness to spend some time?' This is the beginning phase of 'being there' and obviously should be reflected in the eyes of a carer, who is able to position themself in such a way as to look in the same direction as the patient. This will allow both patient and nurse to feel safe in their exchanges, as it allows for eye contact to be disengaged in 'time out', without implying disinterest. Admittedly there are times when cultural differences might deter such practices. Many Aboriginal patients, for example, will usually prefer to look down at the floor if the nurse has not been known to them for a considerable period of time, usually due to shyness rather than disinterest.

Equally, there are many occasions when patients will convey to the nurse their concerns, not with words, but with their eyes. Such expressions can include 'Can I trust you?' 'Do you care?' 'I'm fearful/afraid.' An illustration of this was when an extremely ill patient and a few close relatives all turned their heads at the arrival of a nurse into the room. It was apparent to all present that the nurse was unprepared to 'be there'; this was made clear by the nurse's immediate departure from the room following eye contact between the nurse, the patient and the family members. It is not usual either, for eye contact to be made in isolation of other skills, such as the use of touch. The more obvious communication techniques, however, are usually by use of verbal skills (Stoter, 1995).

The use of words is an invaluable tool in any exchange with patients. The success, though, depends greatly on nurse and patient sharing the same meaning of words. Too many nurses come away from an interaction feeling 'very professional', as they have given of themselves completely; it's sad that the patient may have had great difficulty understanding the nurse's choice of jargon words and colloquial expressions, and may have ended the exchange more confused than at the beginning. It is not just those patients who have a different principal language from the nurse, but also those who have a different socioeconomic background, who belong to a different generation or who have a spiritual/religious background quite different from the nurse. Apart from introducing oneself, a suggested method of commencing the interaction is by demonstrating empathy with the use of an opening statement such as: 'There appears to be something worrying you. I have some time now and would be glad to sit and listen to you.' Should this be acceptable, then the nurse can employ open-ended questions to commence the conversation, questions such as: 'How can I help you?' 'What are your feelings about being in hospital/the treatment/being apart from your family?' or statements like: 'It must be worrying for you here, and I suppose you have had a lot of time to think about things.' Whilst these can initiate a conversation, keeping the dialogue going is another matter. One suggestion is, rather than listening only to the what the patient says, try hearing what is not being said. For example, Mary, a young mother of three children, asked the nurse, 'I'm not going to get better, am I?' Rather than say yes or no, the nurse replied, 'You sound a little fearful, are you afraid of dying?' Having received the reply, 'Yes', the nurse admitted she was as well, and added that she did not really know what to say. This provided an opportunity for both patient and nurse to 'begin to share' and to develop a rapport. Often the phrase 'I don't know what to say' can be indicated to the patient by the use of silence. This is not a difficult skill to use, yet it can be extremely effective in 'saying' to the patient, 'Please go on, I'm listening, I just don't know how to reply to you right now.' When Mary proceeded to explain her concerns about her children's future, the nurse held Mary's hand and remained silent, which allowed Mary to complete her story.

Sometimes the use of silence can encourage a patient to continue, simply because the patient feels uncomfortable with silence and will maintain a dialogue as a means of managing the discomfort. Mary's nurse was asked to listen to her own concerns, to admit an inability to provide a verbal answer and, instead, to provide a true presence.

Many nurses have reasonably effective communication skills and would probably be quite able to employ them in facilitating a patient's spiritual needs. It is obviously beyond this chapter to provide an itemised formula concerning the use of specific communication skills, so further directions should be sought and can be found in most of the communication texts that are readily available.

CONCLUSION

The process of providing spiritual support for a person can be very challenging yet equally rewarding for the caregiver. There are times when the exercise has a successful outcome and times when it is not so apparent. Don't give up, for spiritual growth is a never-ending quest and will ultimately provide any nurse with a more satisfying and fulfilling life, in whatever capacity, whether it be work related or in a social context. Meaning in life is not always clear cut, but 'he who has a why to live can bear with almost any how' (Nietzche, in Frankl, 1964:vii).

As a beginning to your own spiritual discovery, try to answer the question: 'Who am I who comes to give care?' Don't be too perturbed if you can't come up with an immediate response, as it is intended to provide you with an ongoing means of personal exploration.

REFERENCES

Birch C (1990): *On Purpose.* Sydney: New South Wales University Press Ltd.

Buckle J (1993): When is holism not complementary. *British Journal of Nursing* 2 15: 744-745.

Burkhardt MA (1989): Spirituality: an analysis of the concept. *Holistic Nursing Practice* 3 3: 69-77

Burnard P (1989): *Counselling Skills for Health Professionals.* London: Chapman and Hall.

Carson V (1989): *Spiritual Dimensions of Nursing Practice.* Philadelphia, Pennsylvania: WB Saunders.

Cassidy S (1988): *Sharing the Darkness.* London: Darton, Longman and Todd.

Diers D (1990): To profess . . . to be a professional. In: Lindeman C and McAthie M (eds) *Nursing Trends and Issues.* Springhouse, Pennsylvania: Springhouse.

Cella DF and Tross S (1986): Psychological adjustment to survival from Hodgkin's disease. *Journal of Consulting and Clinical Psychology* 54: 616-622.

Clark C and Heidenreich T (1995): Spiritual care for the critically ill. *American Journal of Critical Care* 4 1: 77-81.

Doyle D (1992): Have we looked beyond the physical and psychosocial? *Journal of Pain and Symptom Management* 7 5: 302-311.

Fox M (1988): *The Coming of the Cosmic Christ.* Melbourne: Collins Dove.

Frankl V (1964): *Man's Search for Meaning.* London: Hodder and Stoughton.

Fromm E (1974): *The Art of Loving.* New York: Harper and Row Inc.

Goodloe NR and Arreola PM (1992): Spiritual health: out of the closet. *Journal of Health Education* 23 4: 221-226.

Grey A (1994): The spiritual component of palliative care. *Palliative Medicine* 8: 215-221.

Harrington A (1995): Spiritual care: what does it mean to RNs? *Australian Journal of Advanced Nursing* 12 4: 5-14.

Harrison J (1993): Spirituality and nursing practice. *Journal of Clinical Nursing* 2: 211-217.

Limandri BJ and Boyle DW (1978): Instilling hope. *American Journal of Nursing* 78: 79-80.

Mayerhoff M (1972): *On Caring.* New York: Harper and Row Inc.

Millison M and Dudley J (1990): The importance of spirituality in hospice work: a study of hospice professionals. *Hospice Journal* 6 3: 63-78.

Peck S (1978): *The Road Less Travelled: A New Psychology of Love, Traditional Values and Spiritual Love.* London: Arrow Books.

Narayanasamy A (1993): Nurses' awareness and educational preparation in meeting their patients' spiritual needs. *Nurse Education Today* 13: 196-201.

Price JL, Stevens HO, LaBarre MC (1995): Spiritual caregiving in nursing practice. *Journal of Psychosocial Nursing* 33 12: 5-9.

Renetzky L (1979): The fourth dimension: applications to the social services. In: Moberg D (ed.) *Spiritual Well-being: Sociological Perspectives.* Washington: University Press of America.

Ross LA (1993): Spiritual aspects of nursing. *Journal of Advanced Nursing* 19: 439-447.

Ross LA (1995): The spiritual
dimension: its importance to
patient's health, well-being and
quality of life and its
implications for nursing
practice. *International
Journal of Nursing Studies*
32 5: 457-468.

Rumbold BD (1986):
*Hopelessness and Hope:
Pastoral Care in Terminal
Illness.* London: SCM Press Ltd.

Stoter D (1995): *Spiritual
Aspects of Health Care.*
London: Times Mirror
International Publishers Ltd.

Urden LD, Davis JK, Thalan LA
(1992): *Essentials of Critical
Care Nursing.* St Louis,
Missouri: CV Mosby.

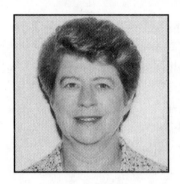

ELIZABETH MACKINLAY
RN, RM, DipNEd, BA, BTh, MEd, FRCNA, doctoral candidate

Reverend Elizabeth MacKinlay, a priest in the Anglican Church of Australia, combines her nurse and priest roles by being a senior lecturer in nursing and a chaplain at the University of Canberra. She is also involved in ministry in a rural parish at weekends. She is married with two adult children.

Over the past fifteen years or so, Elizabeth has developed a special interest in gerontological nursing — assessing the need for education in gerontological nursing, designing and teaching programs and conducting research in the area. More recently she has designed and taught a unit of study in pastoral care and ageing at St Mark's Institute of Theology in Canberra. She has presented numerous papers, seminars and workshops on ageing and spirituality, both in Australia and overseas.

Elizabeth is currently a doctoral candidate at La Trobe University in Melbourne. Her topic is 'Ageing: a spiritual dimension'.

Chapter 6

AGEING, SPIRITUALITY AND THE NURSING ROLE

Gerontological nursing is a complex specialty practice area within nursing. It is at this final stage of the life cycle that really holistic nursing care should be practised. Nurses working in this specialty need a sound basic understanding of the spiritual dimension and ageing in our society to be able to deliver effective nursing care to older adults.

LIVING IN AN AGEING SOCIETY

In Australia, as in most Western countries, we are living in an ageing society. On the one hand, we have many more older people who are in better health than in previous generations and who have much to contribute to society. On the other hand, we have an increasing number of frail older people in the population who require health services. (Even so, only about 5 per cent of older people require long-term residential care.)

Ageing is inevitable, a continual process from birth no matter what people may do to prevent it. But how people age and the possibilities in ageing are not set. In fact, ageing could more properly be described as a social construction; that is, ageing is largely how we see it. If people are able to approach old age with an understanding of the process of ageing and an optimistic outlook, then ageing can be a creative and fulfilling stage of living. If, on the other hand, a person approaches old age with a sense of foreboding, ageing is likely to be far more difficult.

HEALTH ISSUES AND AGEING

Old age is not an illness, it is a part of the life journey. Health issues for older adults have the potential to either add greatly to life satisfaction or to curtail the individual's ability to live independently in the community.

Common myths of ageing may affect the older person's perception of their potential for well-being in ageing, as well as the way health professionals respond to older people. For example, myths related to learning, memory, capacity to work, sexuality and appropriate roles for older people may limit the options offered to older people. Older people themselves will not seek to increase their health status if they are not aware of the possibilities available. Health promotion and the development of effective self-care strategies are an important part of well-being for older adults.

At the same time, extreme old age is often characterised by frailty and increasing vulnerability, with the fear of losing control of bodily functions and of one's mind. Fear of dying, not so much fear of being dead, also looms large for a number of these people (MacKinlay, 1993).

Health in ageing becomes more dependent on holistic functioning of the individual. It is not simply physical health or even psychosocial health but an interrelationship among the physical, psychosocial and spiritual dimensions within each person. In many instances, a decline in physical health may be transcended by the spiritual resources of the individual. In other cases, people who have comparatively better physical health may function poorly through a loss of hope and a loss of the will to go on. Health and illness thus become more complex in the process of ageing.

THE SPIRITUAL DIMENSION IN AGEING

In ageing, the spiritual dimension becomes more important for many. For this discussion, it is important to define spirituality. As it will be used in this chapter, spirituality is:

> . . . that which lies at the core of each person's being, an essential dimension which brings meaning to life. It is acknowledged that spirituality is not constituted only of religious practices, but must be understood more broadly, as relationship with God, however God is perceived by the person, and in relationship with other people (MacKinlay, 1992).

A number of authors have described a decline of interest in religion in older people, based on data that shows a decline in church attendance (organisational religious activity) in old age, particularly in the presence of increasing disability. Ainlay and Smith (1984) and Mindel and Vaughan (1978) in Harris (1990) suggest that decline in attendance at such organisational activities may be offset by an increase in nonorganisational religious activities, including listening to religious radio, watching religious TV, Bible reading and prayer.

Older people's interest and involvement in organisational or formal religious activities may be governed more by availability of opportunities than by lack of interest, particularly in the frail elderly. Thus, studies may show that there is diminished practice of religion by older people when in fact this is not an indication of a lessened importance of spirituality. Rather, it is an indication of a lessened ability to engage in formal religious activities, and a change in emphasis for meeting spiritual needs. For example, private prayer habits seemed to have remained stable for many people (Markides et al., 1987, cited in Schaie and Willis, 1991:333).

SPIRITUAL DEVELOPMENT ACROSS THE LIFE SPAN

Like psychosocial development, spiritual development may continue throughout life. Fowler (1981) developed a life span approach to faith development, maintaining that all humans have a faith dimension in their lives. His definition of faith is very similar to that of spirituality as described by MacKinlay (1992). Fowler maintained that faith develops through a series of identifiable stages across the life span, not unlike the psychosocial developmental theories of Erikson (1968), Piaget (1969) and Kohlberg (1981). However, Fowler's study included few older people, and more research is required to expand the understanding of this final stage of faith/spiritual development.

STAGES OF PSYCHOSOCIAL DEVELOPMENT

Erikson's (1968, 1986) stages of psychosocial development across the life span are central to understanding the link between the psychosocial and the spiritual. His concept of integrity versus despair, in the final developmental stage of ageing, seems to correctly accept the assumption that a task of ageing is to make sense of this life and our part in it. This task has a strong spiritual basis. A number of authors have also observed this relationship, in particular, Kimble (1990:124). Erikson classified wisdom as an important outcome of the final developmental stage of ageing.

I would have to say that, although Erikson classified the final stage of the human life cycle development (integrity/despair) as a psychological dimension, I believe that the spiritual underlies this concept. It is interesting to note that Erikson included material on the spiritual dimension in his book *Vital Involvement in Old Age*, written when he was in his 80s (Erikson, 1986).

It is very much the person's sense of being right with God and in harmony with other people that brings a sense of integrity to ageing. Associated very closely with this is what the person sees as ultimate meaning in life, that is, the spiritual dimension of life.

LINKS BETWEEN THE PSYCHOSOCIAL AND THE SPIRITUAL IN AGEING

The relationship between the psychosocial and the spiritual dimensions is close. In some instances it is difficult to distinguish between the two. Indeed, it may be asked if it is important to distinguish between the psychosocial and the spiritual. I suggest that, in practice, it is essential to look beneath the presenting behaviours to the root cause in any instance. At first an issue may seem to be psychological in nature, but once the psychological aspect has been dealt with, the problem may still be there. For instance, the problem may appear to be guilt. This may be dealt with using counselling, or perhaps even medication for associated depression, but the guilt may still be present.

Identifying the spiritual needs goes still deeper. An older person may carry guilt for something that happened many years ago. The need may be for forgiveness and reconciliation. Only when these issues have been addressed will the guilt finally be laid to rest, and a sense of peace attained.

THE SPIRITUAL JOURNEY IN AGEING

Spiritual development is seen by Clements (1990:56) as the developmental stage of the fourth quarter of life. Ageing is a spiritual journey. That is to say, while physical decline is an expected part of the ageing process, both spiritual and psychological growth and development continue.

Spiritual matters become accentuated at particular times in people's lives, and for older people there may be many times that they are brought face to face with their own vulnerability and mortality. For some, loss of meaning in life can lead to suicide. In Australia the number of older people who end their lives in suicide is increasing at a greater rate than is youth suicide. In 1991–92, according to figures produced by the Australian Bureau of Statistics, there was a 23 per cent rise in deaths by suicide amongst males aged between 65 and 74 years (Appleby, 1994, cited in Stuart-Smith, 1994). It appears that hope is a vital factor in the will to continue living (Frankl, 1984). Those older people who see no hope in continued living are more likely to turn to suicide as a final solution.

Fischer (1985:4) writes that the older person needs to let go in order to be able to move forward; this she sees as the capacity to affirm life in the face of death. Clements considers early old age a time of potential crisis of meaning. He sees the outcome of this crisis as being conversion, but it is much more common to see stripping of roles and shedding of identity.

Shedding of roles held in middle age, and the losses which commonly occur in ageing, are a necessary part of ageing. These changes can be seen as loss of meaning or loss of identity for the individual. Self-emptying or letting go is a necessary prerequisite for spiritual growth for Christians growing into Christ. Stripping, for some, can be understood as 'a sacramental process . . . that leads to God' (Clements, 1990:61) or sometimes simply to an inner emptiness. The stripping away includes roles and cultural and social values learned and practised in earlier years; it may be a painful means of gaining spiritual maturity for some older people. The revealed emptiness at the core of the person's being, without the trappings of society, may be a stark nakedness. This may well stimulate the movement of the individual from doing into being. This may be a time where the older person struggles to relinquish past roles (things she or he may no longer be capable of doing) and comes to an acceptance of God in his or her life. This last stage seems to be reaching a connectedness with God and preparing for 'going home'.

THE SIGNIFICANCE OF REMINISCENCE: A DEVELOPMENTAL TASK OF AGEING

Meaning-making is a part of ageing allied to the concept of wisdom, well known in both Old Testament and New Testament times, but long neglected in Western society.

A part of meaning-making in ageing is associated with reminiscence which occurs naturally for many older people.

Reminiscence is not simply an enjoyable pastime for older adults, but a means to achieving the developmental task of ageing — spiritual maturity. Older people can benefit from guided reminiscence, in group and individual situations. Spiritual reminiscence can be used in spiritual direction and pastoral counselling to assist older adults to come to realise the ultimate meaning of their lives. Kimble writes that 'Memory reveals God's presence in our lives. Faith is the recounting of God's love and presence in our journey through time.' (Kimble, 1990, in Seeber 1990:125)

THE NURSING ROLE IN SPIRITUALITY AND AGEING

Recent literature on caring has been moving increasingly towards recognition of the spiritual as addressed in the dimension of caring. Nurses will readily acknowledge the caring nature of nursing (Brown, Kitson and McKnight 1992). Even so, caring has not always been seen as spiritual. The caring aspect of nursing has often been described as being 'invisible' and, at best, is difficult to quantify.

The spiritual dimension is, I believe, that very component of nursing that nurses seek to discover for themselves in the concept of caring. The spiritual is the component that gives the nurse so much satisfaction in the practice of nursing. Although the spiritual dimension of nursing has so often been invisible in the past, it is possible to identify this dimension, and to develop intentional strategies to meet patient needs in this area.

Many nurses may feel uncomfortable working in the spiritual dimension. Some suggest working in the spiritual dimension may conflict with their own and patient beliefs.

Interventions in the spiritual dimension may be seen as an invasion of privacy. That religion should not be discussed with patients has been one of the nursing myths of the past. And then there is the perennial objection put forward for not giving spiritual care: nurses don't have time.

CHANGES IN NURSING PRACTICE

The recent changes in length of bed stay, resulting in shorter hospital stays combined with increased use of high technology in acute health care agencies, have implications for care of older adults. Being a patient in high technology acute care settings can be confusing for ill older adults (or for anyone for that matter). Acknowledging the human being in the midst of the technology and providing appropriate spiritual care is a real challenge to nurses. Patients are treated and discharged so rapidly that new thinking has to be used to maximise the quality of the caring relationship developed in the time available. The clinical pastoral education model, used widely in clergy and pastoral carer training, is a good one for nurses to follow. Nurses need to learn to connect quickly and deeply with patients to discover the key issues needing attention. Nurses who are effective in providing spiritual care bring their whole selves into the caring relationship, connecting deeply at the spiritual level with those they care for.

In long-term care the quality of relationship between elderly residents and nurses is critical. The nursing relationship and the relationship with other people in the resident's immediate environment can make the difference between the elderly person retaining a sense of integrity in this setting or declining into a state of despair.

SPIRITUAL CARE IS DIFFERENT FROM PSYCHOSCIAL CARE

Psychological and spiritual needs may appear to be very similar, and in fact Highfield (1981, 1992) found in a study of oncology nurses that these nurses often identified spiritual needs as psychological. The problem lies then in using nursing interventions to meet the psychological needs, but failing to address the spiritual dimension. Some of these spiritual issues may be grief, guilt, anger, anxiety, depression, fear, the need to receive and to express love, the need for reconciliation with God and in human relationships, and coming to terms with diagnosis and living with terminal illness.

Admission to a nursing home is a critical time, for few residents return to independent living after residing in a nursing home. One elderly woman told me, 'If I have to go to live in a nursing home I will die.' This woman struggled to maintain her independence in very precarious conditions. She hoped never to go to a nursing home, and indeed she died having remained at home until about a week prior to her death.

Residents of nursing homes certainly do experience a number of spiritual needs and there are many opportunities to assist them to address these needs effectively if the needs are first correctly identified as spiritual needs. These needs are unlikely to all be met by clergy, or pastoral carers, due often to their not being present at the time of need. The obvious group who have the potential to be able to provide spiritual care are the nurses. Yet nurses need first to be convinced of what spiritual care looks like before they are willing to take it on board as part of nursing practice.

SPIRITUAL NEEDS ASSESSMENT

There have been a number of assessment instruments designed to assess the spiritual needs of patients since Ruth Stoll's work in 1979. A pilot study conducted (MacKinlay, 1992) using Stoll's guide, to assess the spiritual needs of older adults, failed to elicit worthwhile information. The questions were too broad and failed to tap into the spiritual needs of the older people. A literature review revealed the most appropriate assessment tool available then, for use with older adults, was the Spiritual Health Inventory (SHI) of Highfield (1981, 1989, 1992) constructed particularly for patients with cancer. This questionnaire was used in a study to assess the spiritual needs of elderly residents of nursing homes (MacKinlay, 1992). Factor analysis revealed four major factors which accounted for most of the variance. The factors were hope, distress of the human spirit, acceptance of God and others, and involvement in life. A new Spiritual Health Inventory, Elderly, (SHIE) was constructed (currently being evaluated) using fewer questions, and focusing on items found to be more critical to older people. Having fewer questions than the original questionnaire, it is more readily used with frail older people with low energy levels. This new SHIE is currently being used in doctoral studies. More work remains to be done in this important area.

When assessing the spiritual needs of an older person, it is vital that nurses first acknowledge their own spirituality, and are thus able to identify and meet the person at the person's point of need. If we are not first sensitised to our own way of being spiritual, it is too easy to project our own needs onto others. Spiritually sensitised nurses, whatever their religious background, will be more able to meet spiritual needs of others, at least to the level of being able to identify them and refer the frail older person to appropriate pastoral care.

SPIRITUAL NEEDS OF FRAIL OLDER ADULTS

Frail older adults often have particular spiritual needs which may or may not be related to religious practices. Sometimes it is the need for forgiveness, or reconciliation with family members, or there may be issues of grief, guilt, resentment, or even anger that emerge for a number of older people approaching the end of their lives.

Loss of control over their life situation and loss of meaning in life can precipitate spiritual crises for frail older people. One older person I cared for experienced spiritual distress due to her incontinence. For her, it was much more than embarrassment, it bordered on shame, that she should have lost such bodily control. We were able to help her by dealing with her incontinence with sensitivity, and connecting with her in respect and love for her as a human being, of value in God's sight.

Assessment of the spiritual needs of frail older adults forms an important part of nursing practice. In research done on spiritual wellness of residents in nursing homes from 1992 to 1994, in Canberra and surrounding areas of New South Wales (reported in part in MacKinlay, 1992), it became apparent that frail elderly residents of nursing homes had many spiritual needs. Anecdotal information arising from interviews with nursing home residents in this study gives some insight into the concerns of these older people. Comments from the elderly themselves varied a great deal. One resident expressed the idea that the nursing home was the 'waiting room for Heaven'.

Another said, 'Not even God could help me now I am in a nursing home, I would rather be dead than here, I would welcome death.' Yet another patient wondered why she had to suffer like this now, and for how long.

Being old and believing that nothing can be done to help formed an important theme for some of those interviewed. These people were residents in a very pleasant environment in very well-run nursing homes. It is apparent that it is not only the environment that is important to these elderly people. Nursing homes are rightly called by some, 'God's waiting room'. Loss of independence in itself reinforces the individual's sense of vulnerability. Needing to depend on others to go to the toilet, to eat, to dress are associated with this sense of loss of control.

Some residents spoke of their faith: 'I must have been kept for some purpose, but I don't know what.' In one woman's response, acceptance of her stage of life is evident as she says, 'I think I have nothing to live for, but I can still enjoy it.' This person also said she thinks about life after death, knowing it will be good. The faith of another elderly woman allowed her to accept being in a nursing home. One person stated that she was fearful about life after death 'because it was so uncertain'. This same person stated she had a strong belief in God, but did not think a minister would understand her fear about life after death. Another resident expressed strong disappointment that there was no contact with a minister of her own denomination at the nursing home. The nursing student involved in this study was able to make this arrangement, which was the beginning of regular contact for this woman with her minister (MacKinlay, 1992).

Death is a subject not often spoken of in a lot of nursing homes. Staff in this study often felt reluctant to introduce the topic. Yet, it is a topic many of the frail residents wanted to talk about.

A factor identified by a number of the registered nurses working in nursing homes was their lack of preparation to address spiritual needs. A number of these nurses were involved in the data-collecting process using the SHI developed by Highfield (1981, 1989) to assess spiritual health. At first the nurses were reluctant to ask some of the questions in the SHI; they said the questions were too invasive and too personal. The SHI asked questions about hope, religion, fears and meaning in life.

Following questions and discussion in the classroom the students felt comfortable about giving the SHI a go in practice. The feedback from the students proved to be one of the most exciting parts of the study. Comments came back such as: 'I had nursed Mrs B. for months, but I never knew these things about her'; 'Once I started asking the questions, it was like opening the floodgates'; 'I found that [after this experience] I changed the way I gave care.'

ASSISTING OLDER ADULTS TO CONTINUE THEIR SPIRITUAL JOURNEY

Nurses can make a valuable contribution to facilitating the spiritual journey of older adults. First, nurses may assist in the reminiscence process. Secondly, nurses may raise community awareness of the potential problems of social and spiritual isolation and facilitate the social and spiritual well-being of older adults. Thirdly, nurses may also use spiritual care to contribute effectively to the quality of life for people who have dementia.

Reminiscence/life review

While life review is a naturally occurring phenomenon in older adults, ways of assisting them to continue and deepen their spiritual journey may be beneficial to many, particularly those with spiritual despair — the spiritual journey should continue until death. In a sense there is a real role here for nurses who work with frail older people — that of meaning-maker. The nurse as meaning-maker may facilitate life review with older adults. Being listened to and assisted to put together the picture of family and the ultimate meaning of all the threads of life are of the greatest importance for those in the last stages of life.

Issues of relationship with God and relationships with others may all be addressed; how guilt is handled, how repentance and forgiveness are experienced are all relevant. These are important issues for the older person coming to an ultimate understanding of their life journey.

Identifying and dealing with social and spiritual isolation

The effects of social and spiritual isolation on frail older adults living alone and housebound are issues which challenge our rapidly ageing society. Meaningful relationships with others are an important part of spiritual well-being.

Recent government trends in Australia have focused on providing more services to older adults in their own homes in an attempt to minimise admissions of older people to long-term care facilities. One aspect of care that is hard to provide for this group of housebound people is the need for a regular intimate relationship with another human being.

Many services for housebound frail elderly people are provided within a tight time frame, making it difficult for those who deliver services, such as meals, to be able to provide any pastoral support while delivering their services.

The effects of this are seen, in some instances, when frail older people deteriorate mentally, having no meaningful contact with other adults from one week to the next. Often family live in distant towns or cities, and there is no-one to transport or visit these people. It is no wonder that depression is often diagnosed in frail older people. In one North American study, 40 per cent of older patients hospitalised with another diagnosis were found to be depressed (Koenig in Kimble et al. 1995:14-15).

Community health nurses have an important role in the care of housebound frail older people, in assessing spiritual needs, making appropriate connections with these older people, and creatively using various resources such as visitor programs.

Meeting the spiritual needs of people who have dementia

Assessing and meeting the spiritual needs of people who have dementia is a specially challenging aspect of care. Often it is possible to connect with people who have dementia through the spiritual, through use of religious services, prayer, Holy Communion and singing. It is important to have a knowledge of any particular religious symbols or rituals the person has been familiar with.

CONCLUSION: PASTORAL CARE, SPIRITUAL CARE AND AGEING

Spiritual care is a part of holistic care, care that is particularly important for frail older people. Whose role is it? Clergy would seem to have a special role here, yet many clergy have had little preparation in their training on caring for older people. For some clergy, the sacraments may form the main part of their work with residents of nursing homes, for others there is a much wider recognition of the scope of spirituality, that may include aspects of pastoral care and counselling.

Nurses are beginning to recognise that the spiritual dimension lies at the very heart of what nursing is. Nursing patients holistically must include the spiritual. Spirituality in ageing is a special part of this. It is a privilege to be able to work with older people, helping them to come to their final and ultimate meanings in this life, meeting them at their point of need, in grief, in loss, in remembering the joys of years gone by, supporting them in their times of pain and suffering.

REFERENCES

Ainlay and Smith (1984): In: Harris DK (1990): *Sociology of Aging*. New York: Harper and Rowe.

Brown JM, Kitson AL, McKnight TJ (1992): *Challenges in Caring: Explorations in Nursing and Ethics*. London: Chapman and Hall.

Clements WM (1990): Spiritual development in the fourth quarter of life. In: Seeber JJ (ed.) *Spiritual Maturity in the Later Years*. New York: The Haworth Press.

Erikson EH, Erikson JM, Kivnick HQ (1986): *Vital Involvement in Old Age*. New York: WW Norton & Co.

Fischer K (1985): *Winter Grace: Spirituality for the Later Years*. New York: Paulist Press.

Fowler JW (1981): *Stages of Faith*. Blackburn, Victoria, Australia: Dove Publications.

Frankl VE (1984): *Man's Search for Meaning*. New York: Washington Square Press.

Harris DK (1990): *Sociology of Aging*. New York: Harper and Rowe.

Highfield MF (1981): Oncology nurses' awareness of their patients' spiritual needs and problems. Unpublished thesis. Little Rock, Arkansas: University of AR for Medical Sciences.

Highfield MF (1989): The spiritual health of oncology patients: a comparison of nurse and patient perceptions. Unpublished dissertation. Denton, Texas: Texas Woman's University.

Highfield MF (1992): Spiritual health of oncology patients. Nurse and patient perspectives. *Cancer Nursing* 15 1: 1-8.

Kimble MA, McFadden SH, Ellor JW, Seeber JJ (eds) (1995): *Aging, Spirituality , and*

Religion: A Handbook. Minneapolis, Minnesota: Augsburg Fortress Press.

Kimble MA (1990): Aging and the search for meaning. In: Seeber JJ (ed.) *Spiritual Maturity in the Later Years.* New York: The Haworth Press.

MacKinlay EB (1992): Spiritual needs of the elderly residents of nursing homes. Unpublished report submitted in part fulfilment of requirements for BTh at St Mark's National Theological Centre, Canberra.

MacKinlay EB (1993): Spirituality and ageing: bringing meaning to life. *St Mark's Review* Spring, 155: 26-30.

Mindel and Vaughan (1978). In: Harris DK (1990): *Sociology of Aging.* New York: Harper and Rowe.

Piaget J (1969): *The Psychology of the Child.* London: Routledge and Kegan Paul.

Schaie KW and Willis SL (1991): *Adult Development and Aging.* New York: Harper Collins.

Stoll RI (1979): Guidelines for spiritual assessment. *American Journal of Nursing* 1574-1577.

Stuart-Smith P (1993): Suicide in the nineties — ethical and pastoral care issues and responses. Unpublished paper submitted as part fulfilment for BTh at St Mark's National Theological Centre, Canberra.

OTHER READING

Highfield MF and Cason C (1983): Spiritual needs of patients: are they recognized? *Cancer Nursing* June: 187-192.

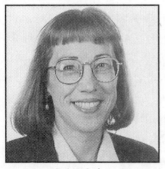

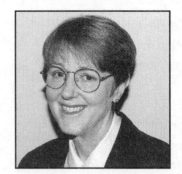

Dr Irene Coulson

Professor Sue Ronaldson

DR IRENE COULSON
RN, BScN, MSAHealth, PhD

Irene Coulson is the Associate Professor in Nursing and Gerontology at the University of New England in New South Wales, Australia. She has many years of experience in research, education, clinical practice, and working with families and persons with dementia in Canada and Australia. She has a special interest in the spiritual care of families and persons suffering from dementia.

Irene has developed the Total Environment Quality of Care Model which provides guidance in the way in which carers interact with residents, demonstrates how the physical environment is laid out and identifies the need to assess how available are support systems in dementia care units. Irene has published and presented, nationally and internationally, her work on people in the latter stages of dementia and improving environments in dementia care units.

PROFESSOR SUE RONALDSON
RN, DipNEd, BSc(Hons), PhD, FRCNA

Sue Ronaldson is Foundation Chair in Nursing of Australian Catholic University and St Vincent's Health Care Campus, Darlinghurst (Sacred Heart Hospice, St Vincent's Hospital and St Vincent's Private Hospital), in Sydney. Sue has established the Nursing Research Unit located at St Vincent's Health Care Campus. She has a long-standing interest and much experience in working with nurses in aged-care facilities. Sue has a particular interest in nurses' caring approaches to addressing psychosocial and spiritual needs of older people living with dementia in long-term care settings. She has published in this area and has frequently consulted and provided education on nursing care of people with dementia. In recent times this consultation has extended to nursing assessment and management of people with AIDS Dementia Complex.

Chapter 7

SPIRITUAL CARE IN DEMENTIA — NURTURING THE HUMAN SPIRIT

THE JOURNEY CONTINUES — SPIRITUAL CARE IN DEMENTIA

Older people who have dementia present a challenge to gerontic nurses in their endeavours to consistently provide quality care. The realities of these people and their carers are often in opposition. These people live in a world which is extracted from their environment. Their behaviours are difficult to understand and their sense of logic is lost. The person with dementia may be confused in a temporal sense, often reliving roles they held previously. They may speak and act in ways that are unintelligible. The here and now reality has little or no meaning to them. In the extreme they may be totally withdrawn, both physically and psychologically. How then can the gerontic nurse assess their spiritual needs?

In order to provide quality care there needs to be some understanding of the person's sense of reality. This reality can be detected through their behaviours and understood within the context of their whole life. Their spiritual being can be seen at times when least expected. They may hold on tightly to people, objects or events which mean something to them that is not immediately obvious to their carers, family or friends.

The gerontic nurse needs to explore these cues in search of an understanding of the person's life meaning. At these times spirituality can be the only thing that is central to their life; what they feel and remember are elements of that spiritual self. No interaction can be left unexplored. While seemingly trivial or unimportant, their cues and interactions hold the key to providing spiritual care — to supporting the personhood, their self.

PERSONHOOD IN DEMENTIA

The spiritual dimension of self has many appropriate definitions. Most include statements which relate to meanings of one's life, purpose and fulfilment in life, the need for hope, and the need to believe in self and in others, as well as having a relationship with a power beyond self (Ross, 1994:33).

Personhood is concerned with being recognised as a person. This desire is so strong that it is maintained throughout the lifespan. The loss of personhood can be minimal if the nurse promotes nursing care that recognises the person's unique characteristics and attributes. Components of personhood include wholeness, being, peacefulness, joyfulness, contentment, self-worth, self-esteem, social aspects, spiritual dimensions, cultural orientation and reality orientation (Bahr, 1992).

Dementia alters a person's ability to remember and to communicate effectively. It is said to also alter personality. However, a person's sense of self is not necessarily dependant on memory and the ability to communicate. People close to a person living with dementia are heard to say: 'She's not the same person as she was', 'This is not the person I married', and 'My wife died when she got this disease'. Family carers are often confused and angry at the changes that have taken place in their loved one. They find it extremely difficult to reconcile the person now with the one before the onset of dementia. They experience a great sense of loss: loss of an identity they knew so well, loss of the opportunity to relate and recall past memories, and loss of the ability to communicate with their loved one and to convey their present distress regarding the effect of the person's disease on their lives.

However, the person with dementia still lives. Can this disease totally rob them of themselves? Some of their spontaneous behaviours suggest not — they suggest that an inner self still exists but only rarely surfaces. Sometimes this may be seen in a once-familiar look, a purposeful walk, or a characteristic gesture.

On this point McGregor and Bell ask a poignant question: 'Does our personality and the sense of awareness of ourselves as a unique and individual human being (the phenomenal self) depend on having a good memory?' (McGregor and Bell, 1993:29). Even though communication is limited in people with cognitive impairment, the spirit or soul can still be connected with in meaningful ways. 'The soul is the self' and according to Hebrew interpretation for the word soul it is 'the deepest life forces that course through every human being' (Everitt, 1996:29-30).

It is important to recognise that memory does not just record events; it is the seat of 'ideas, affection, friendships, likes and dislikes, desires and aspirations' (McGregor and Bell, 1993:28). By limiting our concept of memory to event recall carers overlook the deeper elements of living and the important constructs which give meaning to life. If a person can relive a joyous occasion of old, or a place where once they were happy, then they still have the ability to remember. It is our perception of what is memory that needs to be reshaped in order to revision the lives of people with dementia. This requires a change in mental set, which people may not be prepared for; more often they do not recognise the potential for liberation and restructure of the role of carer. O'Connor suggests there is a need for three paradigm shifts: 'a different way of thinking; a different way of relating; and a different way of using symbols' (O'Connor, 1992, cited in Everitt, 1996:34).

'People often ostracise those with dementia because of the difficulty of maintaining human solidarity with those who are losing their sense of personal identity and their ability to remember' (Everitt, 1996:25). By encouraging people living with dementia to be individuals — to express their needs, wants, emotions and feelings — the stage is set for establishing trusting relationships based on genuine respect of each person's sense of self. Jevne in her book *It All Begins with Hope* makes a strong statement in regard to the need to investigate the full depth of the caring role which is no less relevant when caring for people with dementia: 'I have a vision that caregivers would touch patients, gently and not just physically. That all would recognise that with every touch, every smile, every word, we are entering a temple' (Jevne, 1991, cited in Everitt, 1996:33-34). The sacredness of the soul is each person's temple, which is no less true in people living with dementia.

MOMENTS OF CLARITY — NURTURING THE MIND, BODY AND SOUL IN DEMENTIA

The profession of nursing is committed to providing total care — biopsychosocial care. Most often physical care is provided foremost as it demands attention that is quite obvious. The experienced nurse also readily recognises a person's other needs and their interrelatedness to total well-being. When the mind's capacity is diminished, as in dementia, it is quite difficult to assess needs in this domain.

However, people with dementia may often experience moments of clarity which can be expressed in words but may be also visible in behaviours or emotions expressed. The nurse can tune into the person's spiritual needs in these moments of clarity. If they go undetected the older person with dementia will feel even more lost and alone.

Everitt (1996) describes these moments of clarity as episodes of awakening, specifically spiritual awakening. 'If the definition of a developing spirituality is being open to possibilities, even those with severe dementia can experience, in some unpredictable precious moments, the essence of life — that is, the life force or the spiritual' (Everitt, 1996:31-32). Awakening is a universal spiritual experience. In moments of clarity the person with dementia is briefly experiencing the present moment; they 'experience the numinous in a mysterious way. These times of profound engagement with life challenge us, as caregivers, to appreciate the importance of the present moment in our lives' (Everitt, 1996:32).

The care required during these moments of clarity needs to be focused specifically on the cues given at the time. If a person shakes their head and says: 'I'm lost here' they may mean that for that instant in time they realise that they no longer have control over their life. The use of exploratory nonconfronting questions can help the nurse explore the feelings behind the words. For example, 'You feel lost?',

'Where are you lost?' or simply 'What does it feel like to be lost?'. While the person may not be able to answer any of these questions, your words tell them that you have heard, and that you are concerned about what they have said (Ronaldson and McLaren, 1991; Ronaldson and Savy, 1991, 1992).

People with dementia often express a need to go home — home as a place which is familiar, a place where they once felt safe. 'Home' is a symbol of security and of love and identity — all things that they do not feel now. Nurses can explore what home means to a person, the memories that home evokes and the familiar and loving people they can no longer remember. No matter what or where we call home it is generally a basic ingredient to the lives of all people. Moments of clarity need to be documented so that all carers are aware that the person with dementia still remembers certain elements of life, both present and past.

TENDER, LOVING CARE: THE ROLE OF THE NURSE

Promoting spirituality for persons with dementia is a challenge for nurses due to the loss of health, memory, judgement, reasoning and communication. For many years, spiritual health has been regarded as a personal and private area because it often relates to specific religious practices. Although research continues to speak of spirituality as a medium for coping with stressful experiences and providing coping strategies many researchers state that there is a need to identify how spirituality can be integrated into nursing care (Miller, 1983; Koenig, George and Siegler 1988; Mull, Cox and Sullivan 1987; Bearon and Koenig 1990; Pressman et al., 1990). There is increasing impetus to understand how the nurse plays a vital role in promoting spirituality and health of those afflicted with dementia. Health, as described by the World Health Organisation, is the extent to which people are able to grasp their hope, to satisfy their needs and to change or cope with their environment.

There is an increased focus on spiritual healing as a forerunner to emotional and physical healing and there are lessons for spiritual health as we move to a more sensitive holistic model (Catholic Health Association of Canada, 1994). Some of these are that resentment, anger, affirmation, social support and a positive outlook have a beneficial effect on the healing process. There is no known cure for Alzheimer's disease and many other dementias, however, the nurse who promotes a positive outlook in day-to-day activities promotes spiritual wellness.

There is little written about the role of nurse in the holistic health care model and its impact on spiritual health in dementia. Holistic health is based on the idea that the body, mind and spirit are interdependent and that neglect of spiritual health can impede physical and emotional well-being (Young, 1993; Heriot, 1992). 'The body, mind and spirit are the basics of being human' (Heriot, 1992:22). Reed (1992) states that the components of spirituality include hope, life experiences, religious behaviours, giving and receiving love and meaning and purpose in life.

It is important that the nurse explore with the client the agitation or anger experienced in order to promote daily an inner sense of peace. There is a vital relationship between spirituality and health and susceptibility to illness. Spirituality is central to a person's well-being and it cannot be separated from the physical deterioration the person experiences with dementia. The nurse who provides care and compassion for a person with dementia creates opportunities to explore a religious component, a meaning of life component and a sense of inner peace and hope during years of suffering. Kozier, Erb and Blais (1992:520) state that spiritual well-being is:

> A way of living, a lifestyle that views and lives life as purposeful and pleasurable, that seeks out life-sustaining and life-enriching options to be chosen freely at every opportunity, and that sinks its roots deeply into spiritual values and/or specific religious beliefs.

SPIRITUAL ASSESSMENT AND THE MEANING OF HOPE

Persons with dementia, whether they reside in their home or in nursing homes, continue in life through their spiritual journey, exploring past, present and future events, mitigated by their level of cognitive impairment. The nurse assesses how the person with dementia seeks pleasurable and life-enriching experiences based on their value and belief system.

The role of the nurse is to assess the person's spiritual needs and, based on the assessment, to plan and implement the client's care then evaluate the client's reaction to that care. It is critical that this assessment is based on the client's perception of the world. If there is moderate cognitive impairment the assessment may require several days to complete. A spiritual care assessment requires a person-centred approach and the nurse must make a concerted effort to understand the client's past, their interests, hobbies and spiritual well-being. The major role of the nurse in providing spiritual care is to assess the client's level of hope, meaning and purpose in life.

Hope is an important component of spirituality and is essential in all human beings, especially if illness is present. Hope is closely related to spirituality, relationships with others, achieving health, having positive emotions, anticipating the future, being in a special place and experiencing special moments (Gaskin, 1995). The literature supports that the 'degree of hope a person possesses has been associated with caring relationships, not only relationships with significant others, but also with health care professionals' (Forbes and Hope, 1994:5). In dementia, hope becomes the present with some remembrance of past events. Assessing hope in dementia identifies what is meaningful to the person and then planning care that fosters hope. People with dementia can have lucid moments where they may see through a window of time and ask about the future. For example, one person in the latter stages of dementia stated, 'If I don't get out [discharged from the nursing home] I will die'. Within three months the lady died. The nurse felt that there was a recognition that she knew she would die soon.

People with dementia retain the ability to express their hope late into the dementing process. These moments of hope are often expressed in short sentences or through behaviour. The future to a person with dementia may be the next moment. However small, time remains an important part of the future. For example, one resident in a nursing home stated that an important aspect in life was to continue to have friends. The nurse ensured that the resident sat with her friends at meals and during activities, interacting with her friends, smiling and laughing with them. This activity gave her energy and promoted spiritual well-being. In dementia, hope has often been expressed as hoping to have the continuance of friends and family, hope of a satisfying meal, hope of a comfortable moment, hope of achieving a sense of inner peace.

Spiritual care in dementia provides hope that the person's expectations and needs will be met moment by moment. Hope, an important component of spirituality, has been described as a human response at the core of human life (Forbes, 1994). Hope generates energy and assists the person with dementia to achieve quality of life experiences. For example, one person with dementia suffering from arthritis stated that she hoped and prayed to be comfortable while she resided in the nursing home. The nurses ensured that she was pain free.

The nurse must assess the degree of hope and what aspects the person hopes to achieve in their day-to-day activities. The nurse can assess hope through effective communication techniques and by promoting an atmosphere and environment of relaxation in which hope and trust can be expressed. Various techniques, including reminiscence, relaxation, aromatherapy, music, prayer and symbols, can be used to assist the client to relax and communicate. It is imperative that the nurse listen to the person's words, utterances and nonverbal communication, even if they seem to make no sense. An approach that utilises touch can promote expression of feelings and ideas. The nurse must remain patient and reach out to develop a trusting relationship.

Losses in dementia can be experienced over and over and can leave the person feeling guilty, agitated and angry. Past losses to the person with dementia are as real as if they happened today. Hope is then difficult to maintain. The family and other close relationships, such as nurses, are a source of comfort and it is important to include significant people in planning and integrating care. Families provide a wealth of knowledge about the client and can assist nurses in understanding the client's feeling and ideas. Families can respond lovingly to feelings and are aware of the losses that their loved one has experienced throughout life. The nurse must acknowledge the loss with the client in order to understand their spiritual needs. Everitt (1996) supports that improving the client's spiritual well-being is empowering and provides a sense of inner peace.

The nurse plays an important role in which hope, life experiences, religious behaviours, giving and receiving love and meaning and purpose in life should be explored with the client and family. The spiritual assessment plays an important part in understanding the client's hope, meaning and purpose in life. As well, the nurse assists the person in accepting losses experienced throughout life. By improving spiritual health the client may be able to accept with peace each moment as it arises.

COPING WITH GRIEF AND LOSS

People with dementia experience losses as a result of ageing, as well as those from the dementia. People with dementia experience a multitude of losses that include a loss in health, memory, reasoning, judgement, hope, self-esteem, sense of worth, home, possessions and personhood. These losses can lead to depression, especially in the early stages of dementia. As a nurse it is important to understand the grieving process and its impact on the person with dementia and on the family.

The symptoms of grief may include anxiety, depression, anger, loss of appetite, weight loss, headaches, vomiting, dizziness, skin rashes, chest pain and infection (Kozier et al., 1995). Grief reactions can occur even if the person is reliving a life experience. People with dementia may grieve a loss, such as the death of their mother, as though it happened yesterday. The notion of time in dementia is altered and the person is not always able to consider the future, only the past and present, due to cognitive impairment. By unlocking memories, we connect to the human spirit and assist the client through their spiritual journey. Everitt (1996:85) describes time for the person with dementia:

> For those of us who are cognitively intact, time is like a stream of water in which we float with the current. For someone with Alzheimer's disease, time is frozen into individual snowflakes that touch the skin and melt.

People with dementia constantly find themselves tangled in the web of their own minds (Everitt, 1996). It is important that the nurse understand the ideas and feelings that the person is trying to express in their endeavours to resolve the grief and loss experienced. Resolving grief should be one of the major aims when caring for someone with dementia. There is a need for further research in understanding the stages of grief resolution for persons with dementia, and their families, to promote spiritual and physical well-being.

Three stages of grief resolution for a person with dementia have been described by Sandmaier (cited in Everitt, 1996): separation, marginality and reintegration. In separation, the person experiences a separation from the self and their community. The second stage of grief resolution is called marginality and the person feels they no longer have a voice or are not able to participate in a meaningful way. The third stage of grief resolution is 'reintegration and brings a new understanding of the purpose of life with the understanding of the changed identity of the loved one' (Sandmaier, in Everitt 1996:89).

In this chapter Coulson proposes five stages of grief resolution based on clinical experiences with persons with dementia. These stages are desperation, disconnection, anger, depression and images of the twilight. By understanding stages of grief resolution the nurse can assist persons with dementia and their families to successfully cope with the present, therefore promoting improved quality of life.

In the first stage of grief resolution the person experiences desperation. The person with dementia suspects that something is wrong when reasoning and judgement are affected and short-term memory fails. Even though the person suspects that something is not right they may joke about it or ignore the problem. The person continues to cope with life as cognitive impairment continues. The person refuses to accept that something is wrong and tries desperately to carry on with activities of daily living. Friends and loved ones may begin to notice changes in behaviour, such as forgetfulness, and attribute this to other factors.

The second stage is disconnection, where the person senses a disconnection between the body and mind. The person may be physically healthy, however memory, judgement, reasoning and mathematical abilities begin to become noticeably affected. When confronted the person may insist that nothing is wrong, nevertheless, the person becomes aware that intellectual capacity is diminished. The way in which the person views their world begins to change. For example, the person may be aware that they get lost when going for a walk or forget their name when asked. The person may attempt to hide losses by not seeking help or isolating themselves. Eventually loved ones and friends encourage the person to seek help. One person with dementia said that she knew something was wrong since she could feel changes happening daily in her mind but not her body. Often she would awake in the morning screaming from nightmares. She could not differentiate dreams from reality. When asked if she wanted to be told what was wrong she said that she did not. Perhaps the knowledge and impact of the future losses she would experience could not be accepted at this time. There was a sense that the person knew she was dying. The nurses provided support by assisting her to explore her feelings of fear and anxiety. Over time there was an increased sense of spiritual well-being.

In the anger stage the person becomes more aware that something is wrong but, with difficulty, continues to cope with their daily activities. There is an attempt by the person to bring routine, consistency and harmony to their environment. Continued loss of judgement or reasoning, or changes in routine, profoundly upset the person. Loved ones often become frustrated and upset, not knowing what is wrong or what to do. There may be many visits to the doctor, counsellor or minister over a period of months or years to finally come to a diagnosis. Once a diagnosis is obtained, the person may still feel anger due to the losses that have been experienced. Furthermore there may be significant cognitive impairment and loss of verbal communication. The person may be observed to call out, shout, wander aimlessly and become physically and verbally aggressive. These behaviours signal a call for help and it is critical that the nurse develop an understanding of the losses, feelings and ideas that the person is experiencing. As the person continues through life's most difficult journey they seek to improve quality of life in a world that is chaotic.

In the fourth stage, depression, the person may refuse to interact with people and their environment. The journey is lonely and almost unbearable and the person is overwhelmed with loss of structure and quality in life. Time seems endless and the person requires close monitoring to prevent sudden deterioration of health. The person may cry for long periods; they may refuse to eat or participate in activities. When opportunities are provided for participation, the person may withdraw and become isolated. One patient with Alzheimer's disease, living in a nursing home, explained that she felt alone and was depressed because she had an awareness that she was dying. In the depression stage she said that life would never again be happy or productive.

In the fifth stage, called images of the twilight, the person with dementia demonstrates a sense of harmony between self and the environment. Images of the twilight signifies the latter stages of dementia 'where the sufferer is suspended in time, a place of limbo, at the edge of existence' (Breaden and Coulson, 1994:15). How nurses describe this zone offers important insights into the complexity of the world of the dementia sufferer. The person is able to perceive their world in the present and experience the care, touch, and soothing voice of the nurse in an environment that offers acceptance and peace.

The quest for meaning and purpose is central to our existence (Catholic Health Association of Canada, 1994:11) and none of us walks alone on this journey. When the person with dementia is assisted to progress through their journey they may move towards a sense of peace and improved quality of life. The process of achieving spiritual well-being requires the nurse to reach out, listen and respond to the feelings and ideas expressed by the person with dementia. The person living with dementia experiences fear, terror and anxiety in a world they cannot understand. It is critical that the nurse develops an understanding of the losses experienced by the person and works towards assisting them to explore and validate their feelings.

THE USE OF RITUALS, PRAYER AND SYMBOLS

The nurse must gain an understanding of the person's use of rituals, prayers and important symbols that have been used throughout life. Values and beliefs are expressed through behaviours such as rituals and prayer. Questions that address important religious practices, sources of strength, important celebrations, sources of hope and values and beliefs contribute to the development of the spiritual care plan. As well, the nurse should utilise family members who have a wealth of knowledge to assist in gathering data.

It is important that the nurse develops an understanding of the person's history to determine accepted approaches to spiritual care. Families or persons with dementia may become angered if a visit to a priest is arranged and the person is not of the priest's religion. Furthermore, spiritual care encompasses more than support from religious persons but includes the use of rituals, prayer and symbolism.

The use of rituals is effective in promoting spiritual care and provides a sense of rhythm and hope in life. Rituals such as the celebration of birthdays, weddings, anniversaries, Christmas, Easter, attending church, prayer, blessings, administering the sacrament and cultural traditions can evoke emotions and memories (Everitt, 1996). Persons with dementia eventually lose the ability to remember important events, however, when the events are celebrated, their memory of the past is triggered.

For example, the person may think about close relatives that are not present and ask where they are at Christmas. Traditions learned early in life will be remembered because they are deeply embedded in the memories of persons with dementia.

Symbols are another strategy that can be used to promote spirituality and stimulate memory. Symbols that can be used include religious books, a Christmas tree, Easter lilies, a Buddha statue etc. A cross can create peace and solitude. One Christian person with dementia who would not stop shouting was taken to the chapel by the nurse, in the hope that this would calm her. Once in the chapel, she became quiet and pointed to the altar and the cross without saying a word. The nurse stayed, held her hand and prayed with her. The person bowed her head in prayer and later said, 'Amen'. This action provided the person with hope. She seemed to indicate that her needs were being met and she gained renewed energy to continue. The nurse felt that the use of symbols and rituals reminded the woman that God cared for her.

Prayer is an effective strategy that can be used to assist the person to find restored energy and hope to continue on in life's journey. Prayer can transform the experience of illness through hope and love. Touch is often used in prayer, such as anointing with oil. Touching during prayer increases the person's awareness that you are present and both of you are connecting with a higher power.

Prayer can also be performed by reciting verses from a religious book. For example, reciting the 23rd Psalm can be a source of comfort and can trigger fond memories from the past. Eventually the person with dementia may not be able to recite verses from the Bible, but they are able to sing them.

This change in communication occurs as a result of the disease process. Singing church songs or prayers provides another medium in which the person with dementia can express spirituality. For example, a minister who had dementia could verbally communicate in only three- to four-word sentences and eventually became depressed. The nurse discovered that he could sing church songs and lead other residents in hymns. With time, the resident demonstrated renewed strength and purpose in life. Studies show that prayer contributes to health and well-being and is a key factor in promoting spiritual well-being (Catholic Health Association of Canada, 1994).

The use of rituals, symbols and prayer are important strategies to promote spiritual well-being and stimulate memories. It is important that the nurse obtain an accurate history of the person's use of rituals, symbols and prayers. The nurse must promote an atmosphere and environment that will promote the expression of the person's values and beliefs.

DREAMTIME: THE ROLE OF REMINISCENCE

Reminiscing is generally a pleasurable and enjoyable experience for most people. Older people are believed to reminisce more frequently and possibly more openly. Reminiscence helps to contextualise our life, its significant events and relationships. Identity and self-esteem are enhanced by recalling previous roles in life, their successes and failures. Are older people with dementia excluded from this healing activity and can they benefit from the act of reminiscence?

Living in a confused and confusing world people with dementia are at risk of losing their personal identity as they are not able to control their relationship with the world around them.

They may be confused in time and about people, as if they were actually living their reminiscence. They may speak of significant people from their life and misidentify a person close to them. This behaviour may be dismissed as illogical, however, if their behaviours and words are observed and listened to carefully there may be some sense in what they do and say. These people are often uninhibited in their expression, saying things that others would only dare think! These expressions cannot then be discounted as senseless.

Encouraging a person who is confused because of dementia can help the person relive precious moments they themselves cannot recapture. The activity of reminiscing can be carried out in many ways and need not be restricted to a designated time of day. If the person responds positively to reminiscence the carer should endeavour to weave it into the total care approach for a quality environment. If someone experiences strong emotions as a result of reminiscing, this does not necessarily mean a negative outcome. All human beings have stored strong emotions and, given the right trigger, these emotions will be released, often when least expected. Expressions of strong emotions can be a relief and may result in decreased anxiety.

There are many ways to introduce reminiscence into the caring environment. An important start is an awareness of people's personal and social life history. Reminiscence can involve a one-to-one strategic intervention or groups remembering specific social themes or events. It can also involve the use of aroma and music therapies.

Aromas evoke specific memories of occasions long forgotten in all of us. They do the same in some people with dementia. There are aromas that evoke a universal response: for example, those of baking bread or cooking a roast. Not only are these aromas pleasant to experience, they evoke memories of special occasions often associated with home, communal activities and a sense of belonging. These are long-known and readily recognised aromas. The scents of certain flowers, in particular roses, are strong sensory stimuli. It is not uncommon for people to smell the beautiful scent of a rose. Another strong aroma is that of an open wood fire — which stimulates feelings of warmth and security as well as memories of times spent sitting peacefully looking into, and beyond, an open wood fire. For many older people the open wood fire was a common home occurrence also associated with communal activities of gathering and chopping wood, and of building a wood storage heap to make provision for a long winter. A certain pride is also attached to setting a blazing fire and keeping it stoked.

Music is another strong trigger for reminiscing and remembering. Some people with dementia retain the ability to recall the words of songs long after everyday verbal communication is diminished. One elderly man was physically and verbally uncommunicative yet he was able, on a special social occasion, to sing in a beautiful tenor voice, 'Danny Boy', word perfect and full of emotion. His eyes and facial expressions recorded the joy of singing a once-familiar song.

HELPING HUMOUR

It is important when caring for people with dementia that they are not considered to be an homogenous group. Despite cognitive impairment these people have individual differences in behaviour, in personality, in their responses to the environment, and in the way they communicate and let their needs be known. Communication is a central element in any caring relationship; it is very important when caring for people with dementia and it is the nurse's responsibility to facilitate communication.

People differ in their use of humour in their lives. A person's lifelong sense of humour and love of laughter can remain relatively intact in the face of dementia. Encouraging and facilitating humour in these people is a very valuable caring activity. In times of unexpected lucidity a person's humour may shine through. 'The messages that individuals select are based upon the unique past experiences and predispositions of each individual' (Buckwalter et al., 1995:12).

People with dementia can express their individuality through humour and humorous moments. Humour is a vehicle through which they can express themselves in the face of tragic circumstances including declining health. Expressions of humour must be respected and the nurse can take the precious opportunity to laugh too. All caregivers should be encouraged to utilise humour, when appropriate, in a manner acceptable to each individual. 'Therapeutic humour refers to laughing with, rather than at, someone' (Buckwalter et al., 1995:14).

PASTROL CARE AND PARISH NURSING

Meeting the spiritual needs of persons with dementia is the responsibility of families, close friends, nurses and designated chaplains and other religious persons. Hospitals and other care facilities today commonly provide pastoral care services to promote spiritual well-being. The role of pastoral care services in some organisations has expanded to include parish nursing which aims to support religious traditions of people from all faiths; their search for meaning and purpose, love and compassion, forgiveness and hope and their exploration of ethical issues. Historically the church has been involved in important transitions in people's lives that include developmental transitions as well as crisis and situational transitions. A parish nurse is an experienced, university-prepared registered nurse with an advanced understanding of the healing ministry. Pastoral care nurses can provide faith and health-promoting services to religious and nonreligious persons, in the context of strengthening the person in difficult times.

Parish nursing is a new concept that began in the United States and has now spread to other parts of the world. Currently in the United States there are more than 3000 parish nurses (Catholic Health Association of Canada, 1994). Parish nursing is described as the role of a nursing 'member of the parish team who attends to the psychosocial and spiritual wounds of the community' (Simmington, in Catholic Health Association of Canada, 1995:64). Simmington agrees that the parish nurse promotes health as an educator, counsellor, advocate, referral agent and an organiser of parish volunteers. The parish nurse can provide support to persons with dementia and their families and can take responsibility for their spiritual well-being. The parish nurse can provide referrals and education to promote health and spiritual well-being. Families need a competent professional who can counsel, provide information and offer support in a time of need (Coulson, 1993).

There is a need to continue the development of parish nursing within a community and nursing home context. It is imperative that nurses receive education to acquire pastoral care skills and an understanding of spiritual well-being in dementia.

Parish nursing is a process in which the nurse assists persons with dementia and their families to move towards peace and harmony.

THE JOURNEY BEYOND: IMAGES OF THE TWILIGHT

Within the context of spiritual care in nursing, images of twilight conjure up misty half-light, half-dark scenes that suggest the present is related to both its past and its future. For people living with dementia it is a very long, hard and lonely journey. The journey beyond the present can elevate the person's life in terms of their personhood and dignity. This can be achieved through recognition of the existence of their spiritual self by those who care. This is the gerontic nurse's ultimate challenge: to facilitate the journey of each person's self.

Central to this caring role is communication, in all its forms and dimensions. The nurse is fulfilled when listening, observing and touching the soul of each person with dementia; when nurturing the human spirit.

REFERENCES

Bahr RT (1992): Personhood: a theory for gerontological nursing. *Holistic Nurse Practitioner* 7 1: 1-6.

Bearon LB and Koenig HG (1990): Religious cognitions and use of prayer in health and illness. *Gerontologist* 30: 249-253.

Breaden K and Coulson I (1994): Images of the twilight: Alzheimer's disease and palliative care. *American Journal of Alzheimer's Care and Related Disorders and Research* September–October: 15-23.

Buckwalter KC, Gerdner LA, Hall GR, Stolley JM, Kudart P, Ridgeway S (1995): Shining through: the humour and individuality of persons with Alzheimer's disease. *Journal of Gerontological Nursing* March: 11-16.

Catholic Health Association of Canada (1994): *Integrating Health and Values*. Ottawa: Catholic Health Association of Canada.

Coulson I (1993): The impact of the total environment in the care and management of dementia. *American Journal of Alzheimer's Care and Related Disorders and Research* May–June: 18-25.

Everitt D (1996): *Forget Me Not: The Spiritual Care of People with Alzheimer's*. Edmonton. Alberta. Canada: Inkwell Press.

Forbes SB (1994): Hope: An essential human need in the elderly. *Journal of Gerontological Nursing* 20 6: 5-10.

Gaskin S (1995): The meaning of hope: Implications for nursing practice and research. *Journal of Gerontological Nursing* March: 17-24.

Heriot CS (1992: Spirituality and aging. *Holistic Nurse Practitioner* 7 1: 22-30.

Jevne R (1991): *It All Begins with Hope*. Lura Media, San Diego.

Koenig HG, George LK, Siegler IC (1988): The use of religion and other emotional regulating coping strategies among older adults. *Gerontologist* 5 2: 1-11.

Kozier B, Erb G, Blais K (1992): *Fundamentals of Nursing: Concepts, Process and Practice.* USA: Addison-Wesley Company.

Kozier B, Erb G, Blais K, Wilkinson JM (1995): *Fundamentals of Nursing: Concepts, Process and Practice.* 5th edn. Sydney: Benjamin/Cimmings, Penguin Books.

McGregor I and Bell J (1993): Voyage of discovery. *Nursing Times* 89 36: 29-32.

Miller JF (1983): *Coping with Chronic Illness: Overcoming Powerlessness.* Philadelphia: FA Davis.

Mull CS, Cox CL, Sullivan IC (1987): Religion's role in the health and well-being of well-elders. *Public Health Nursing* 4: 151-159.

O'Connor TS (1992): Ministry without a future. *Journal of Pastoral Care* 1 46: 6-10.

Pressman R, Lyons JS, Larson DB, Strain JJ (1990): Religious belief, depression and ambulation status in elderly woman with broken hips. *American Journal of Psychiatry,* 147: 758-760.

Reed PG (1992): An emerging paradigm for the investigation of spirituality in nursing. *Research in Nursing and Health* 15: 349-357

Ronaldson SM and McLaren H (1991): *A Time To Care.* Sydney: High Plains Press.

Ronaldson SM and Savy P (1991): Validation therapy: a viable option for gerontic nursing practice. *Geriaction* Autumn: 7-10.

Ronaldson SM and Savy P (1992): Communication with the confused older person: validation therapy is an option for nursing practice. *Australian Nurses Journal* May: 19-21.

Ross L (1994): Spiritual care: the nurse's role. *Nursing Standard* 8 29: 33.

Young C (1993): Spirituality and the chronically ill Christian elderly. *Geriatric Nursing* November–December: 298-303.

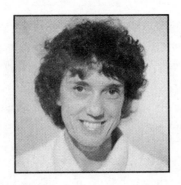

ROSEMARY LANCASTER
RN

Born in England, in the rural county of Herefordshire, Rosemary Lancaster completed her general education at Ross Grammar School. She trained to become a Registered Nurse at King's College Hospital, London, then spent over a year at Preston Hall Chest Hospital in Kent where she gained the British Tuberculosis Association and National Thoracic Surgery certificates. After training and registration as a midwife she went to Zambia in Central Africa, working in Lusaka and Livingstone in general nursing and midwifery.

For over twenty years she has lived in Perth, Western Australia, where she has been employed in several nursing homes. Amongst her qualifications are gerontological nursing, palliative care and basic counselling certificates. As a Christian she worships in the Anglican community and is a licensed pastoral assistant. Her growing revelation of the meaning and the importance of spirituality as a vital component in her personal life has encouraged and equipped her to practise true holistic nursing within her field of employment.

Rosemary is married and has a close family of three daughters and their partners, who live in nearby Perth suburbs.

Chapter 8

THE MEANING OF SPIRITUALITY AND THE NURSE'S ROLE IN PROVIDING SPIRITUAL CARE TO THE DYING PATIENT

One does not live by bread alone.

Bread in this quotation is used in the Biblical way (Deut. 8:3, Matthew 4:4) to mean 'the staff of life' — that food which nourishes and sustains the physical being. So if people are physical beings, and we must surely all agree they are, and if they receive sufficient food and nourishment to maintain their body, why isn't this enough? Why can't we live by bread alone?

It is because human beings are not made up of just a body, they have a mind and a spirit as well.

Historically nurses have been prepared in the medical model, to treat the physical body, or the part of it which is ailing — the fractured femur, or the diseased appendix, the ailing kidney or heart. Little regard was given to the person who owns those parts.

During this century much more emphasis has been given to people's minds than was previously the case. Psychiatrists and psychologists have received greater recognition. Generally, people are not embarrassed to go and see a 'shrink', as they once were derogatively called, and these specialists are welcomed as valuable members of the health care team.

But what of the patient's spiritual dimension? How many nurses give spirituality as much emphasis during the course of their working day as they give to nurturing the bodies and the minds of their patients?

As nurses educated to heal or cure physical illness, we have this as our priority, if not our only role. Even if we have been aware of other facets of healing, we have tended to shy away from them. We feel embarrassed or uncomfortable when patients or their family and friends raise matters concerning spirituality. We may say we have no time, there are already too many tasks to do, and we don't want to get caught up in other issues. In this age of specialisation we see each person as having a specific role, an expertise in a certain area, and therefore we should not encroach on another's particular field. Some nurses may acknowledge a patient's need for spiritual expression, but feel inadequate to deal with it, due to their own lack of training, or their own spiritual doubts. There are others, and probably these are the majority, who are not quite sure what spirituality is.

Many people regard spirituality and religion synonymously. I believe that, whilst the two are related, they are not the same. Religion refers to a person's belief system and their expression of that faith within an organised framework. Certain practices and rituals, such as prayer, worship, and receiving the sacraments, differ according to whether the person is a Christian, a Hindu or a Jew, or belongs to another religion.

The second way of looking at spirituality has separated it from the physical, making it somehow a part of 'another world' thus denying a person's body and humanness.

The third way, the way I will consider it, expresses spirituality in terms of a person's view of the world, or attitude to life. For me, spirituality lies in the heart of a person's being, it is the core, or centre, of their very existence. It is that which gives a person vitality and life, regardless of their belief system or what physical state they are in; what age, sex or race they are; or what social standing they enjoy. Spirituality, then, is that which gives meaning to life. It determines how one views oneself, others and the world around. It is unique to each person and gives an inner harmony and 'wholeness', enabling each of us to transcend external pressures and dilemmas.

Some people, whilst laying no claim to religion, will, in fact, speak of a god, or a force which has a higher power greater than themselves. Great literary artists, including William Wordsworth, recognised a spirit in nature. Painters, such as Michelangelo and Hans Heysen, athletes and many famous musicians have admitted to outpourings of spiritual energy when painting, performing or composing. Taken in this context, just as everyone has a heart, everyone has a spirituality.

My conviction is that each patient must be cared for holistically; that is to say, as nurses, we should nurture not only the body and the mind, but also the spirit. All these components are interactive and each affects the other. To neglect any one will have a deleterious effect on the others.

It is a fact of life that nowadays many people have no religious affiliation or a belief in God. These people may feel they have no spirituality and no need for it, especially when life is good to them. But often when a person is approaching death or has been given a diagnosis of a life-threatening illness, a 'death sentence', they may reconsider their view. For the first time they question their beliefs and the meaning of life. They, in fact, experience a 'spiritual crisis'.

Dr Derek Doyle (1983) states that nearly 75 per cent of dying people will speak of spiritual issues in the last weeks or months of their lives, regardless of their previous beliefs. This is a clear indication that, to the dying person, their spiritual dimension is just as important as their physical and emotional ones.

To whom can the dying person turn in their fear and confusion? Not to their doctor — he or she is too busy. Not to their family — it is not fair to burden them any further. Not to a priest — a priest wouldn't understand their unbelief and would maybe try to force religion on to them, which they do not want. The nurse, however, is seen as available and approachable, so very often they turn to the nurse.

But is the nurse the most suitable person to provide spiritual care to a dying patient? Have we the ability to address another's spiritual needs when we have probably had no educational preparation in this matter?

The answer is 'yes' to both questions. We all possess within ourselves the resources which are necessary to provide spiritual care to another human being. There is no denying that, for some people, their spirituality does lie in their deep belief and personal relationship with God. For these people it may be very important that they continue those practices which provide comfort and support, especially during times of illness. They may need few, or no, other spiritual outlets.

It is the nurse's responsibility, on these occasions, to respect that person's religious needs and assist in whatever way is necessary. It may be appropriate to refer them to a minister of their religion, in order for their faith to be nurtured. As nurses we are not expected to fulfil the duties of a trained minister, but we are required to assist the patient to access one if that is their need.

Nor should we try to introduce our beliefs to another person, if that is not what they want. One person's experience will not provide another's short cuts, nor prevent that person from engaging in their own spiritual struggle. No matter how well-intentioned the nurse may be, at times it is essential to contact a minister of the patient's own faith, showing respect for people of different religions.

But spirituality is not just something to do with religion, it is universal, present in every person, central to everyone's needs, an integral part of their make-up. As Teilhard de Chardin says,

> We are not human beings having a spiritual experience. We are spiritual beings having a human experience (cited in Covey, 1989:319).

When death is approaching there is a special urgency. The patient has a limited future. Time can no longer be taken for granted, there is not much time left. They speed up their striving to find meaning to this life, their searching for a sense of belonging. There are so many questions to ask: Why has this happened to me? Did I do something wrong? What will happen to me when I die? What happens after death, is there another life? They are crying out to have their unconscious selves — their spirit — nurtured.

The dying are compelled to change their focus from being cured to accepting the reality of impending death. They are on their final journey, and it is full of doubts, fears, regrets and loneliness. They are grieving for what has been, what could have been, and for what they will miss in the future. Their fears need to be faced, their doubts, regrets and joys need to be acknowledged and aired.

During this time a patient may explore or re-live their whole life, each event and relationship which has impacted upon them. They experience again the happiness and joy of treasured times, success and people, and the love they have been shown and given. They also pass through the pain of losses, disappointment, failures and rejection, and often they may deal with suppressed aspects of the past. If they reach a stage of acceptance and let go of the pressures, they may have new insights, and get in touch with their true feelings, their needs and desires. All things are put in perspective and they see where they, as a unique and special individual, fit in the universal plan in this constantly changing rhythm of life. With this new understanding, they acquire an inner freedom, a spiritual peace, the healing they have been seeking.

It is important that we, as nurses, do not desert the patient at this stage of their journey. We should be willing to draw near and be there with them and for them. Sometimes it can be the hardest part of all, to just 'be' and not to 'do'. We may have to learn how to move with the patient, not always to respond paternalistically. Whilst at times it is necessary to be a leader and an advocate, at others it may be appropriate for us to follow the patient's lead, to empower them to be in control. A person's need to be in control of their lives does not change when they are approaching death.

The dying person needs a companion, a friend to walk with them, one who will listen, who will share their pain and suffering, who is sensitive to their needs and who assists them to explore and realise their own unique form of spirituality. In order to be this companion it is necessary for the nurse to be comfortable with themselves, to have faced their own fears, especially of illness and suffering, death and dying.

Help is most beneficial to another when given out of the depth of one's own life experiences. At some time in our lives we have all known a sense of failure and feelings of being alone. Most people will also admit to being afraid of dying, so can identify, to a certain extent, with the fears and struggles of the dying person. We are, quite simply, 'in this together', travelling in the same direction. We all share the same humanity, the carers are no better, or wiser or elitist than those they care for.

In order to be of help, it is not necessary for the nurse to have suffered exactly the way the patient is suffering, just as we do not need to have experienced a particular physical illness in order to care for that person. But we need to be sensitive and responsive, affirming their self-worth. We can help to relieve their distress, but we know, as do the patients, that we cannot perform miracles.

It is essential that we move away from the emphasis on competence and the giving of intellectual answers, or counselling. We need to remember that we are there as a bodily presence, in a mutual role, to share in each other's experiences. No special expertise or training is necessary for this role. There are no hours of study to perform or examinations to pass. There is no external determinant of a good friend; only the carer and the cared-for can be the judge.

There are, of course, certain similarities in the ways in which people respond to illness or death. For example, the stages of the 'grief process' are well documented (Kübler-Ross, 1970). To have some knowledge of this may help us avoid distressing reactions to what we would otherwise see as inappropriate behaviour. But we must avoid generalisations, and categorising people, looking instead for their uniqueness and individual responses.

The emphasis in spiritual care lies in relationship, not on knowledge. Carl Rogers (1961) describes this relationship as having 'unconditional positive regard' for another person. The attitude the nurse has, and the interest shown in the patient, will partly determine how willing that patient is to confide in the nurse, share their concerns and ask their questions. When we are privileged to be chosen as the 'listening ears', it is important that we do just that, listen with all our being. Until we learn to listen attentively to another, blocking out our own agendas and need to provide solutions, we will not hear the cries of pain or distress which underlie their stories. We will not be able to respond with empathy, entering with the patient into their fear and confusion, sharing their concerns, their anger and guilt, their search for meaning. By giving someone our full attention we are providing them with spiritual care.

Words can frequently get in the way of caring. There is often more to be gained by being silent, and we should not be afraid of this. The nurse's presence may be all the patient demands. It is not necessary to always be talking; we should not imply that we know all the answers. The dying person needs to be in control and to direct the conversation, the carer responding with openness, honesty and compassion.

It is important that the nurse is sensitive to the patient's need for quietness and time to be alone. This solitude does not necessarily mean that the patient is lonely. They now need time to think and work through life's and death's issues, without the noise, chatter, hustle and bustle that can surround them during daily activities. It is necessary to appreciate their privacy and not to intrude on their wish for silence.

The therapeutic act of touch, simply holding a patient's hand or placing your hand on their shoulder, may do much to alleviate their fears and anxieties, and demonstrates that you care. However, it is important to remember that, for some, touch may be unwelcome, and may even intrude into their private expression of grief.

No dying person will be able to concentrate on their final business unless they are in a calm, comfortable, relaxed atmosphere. It is essential that this is provided and may include the playing of the dying person's choice of music. This music may have special meaning to them, causing memories and emotions to surface, enabling deeper exploration of life's experiences and meaning.

Pain and other distressing symptoms need to be controlled, which may mean calling on allied health professionals or family and friends who have significant meaning to the dying person. No-one who is distressed with physical or emotional problems is able to think or concentrate on life's and death's important issues.

Used correctly, humour and lightheartedness may help to alleviate tension and lighten another person's burden. To see humour in an otherwise unbearable situation may make it somehow acceptable, and may assist the patient in the spiritual healing process. Surrounding a person with beautiful things such as favourite paintings, pleasing decor, plants, and crockery can also be spiritually uplifting.

It is important that the nurse enables the patient to express their feelings of guilt, failure or inadequacy, as well as their anger. There is a need to complete unfinished business and to forgive themselves and others, of perceived as well as actual deeds committed or omitted.

A terminally ill patient may need assistance to work through their grief, as they come to acknowledge that life as they have known it is coming to an end. We must not deny their pain, or their sense of impending loss, but we can be with them as they face reality.

Everything the dying person talks about is important to them and we must not dismiss it lightly. We must also accept the person, as they are and where they are, respecting them and their confidentialities. In this way we affirm their value and self-worth. At times dying patients may ask very difficult questions to which we are not able to help them find answers. They will find peace if they cease to struggle with those questions and are content with the mysteries.

It is vital that a dying person is at all times treated as a valued individual; shown respect and compassion, as well as complete honesty. If the treatment is going to be uncomfortable, or the prognosis is poor, it is important to gently inform the patient of this at an appropriate time. Sooner or later they will realise if the nurse has not been honest, and may no longer feel they can trust that person.

As nurses we must not fall into the trap of being always 'nice' to the dying person. We should be ready to share negative feelings and encourage them to do the same. This will prevent feelings of resentment which may damage the relationship. If we pretend to be what we are not, the patient will often realise this and their anxiety and fear may be increased. By acting falsely we prevent them from feeling accepted and so block their path to healing.

This acceptance of the other person must extend to those we often call 'difficult' or unlovable — the noisy or bad-tempered person, the one who appears unnecessarily demanding or fault-finding. We must resist the temptation to spend longer periods of time with the 'good' or the 'easy' patients, or to try and change the ones we like least into our perceived model of an ideal patient. A severe or life-threatening illness is not the catalyst to change a personality. It is most likely that a person who has been bad-tempered all their life will continue to be this way during a terminal illness.

We must not be condescending or patronising to the patient. Giving them advice or acting as their leader is also to be avoided, as it places us above them. It does not assist them to grapple with their own problems and may stifle legitimate anger or frustration, preventing them from finding their own answers.

Both the nurse and the patient are very vulnerable in this relationship. There is a risk in giving and sharing of ourselves. We may feel a failure when we do not know the answers to difficult questions. We may use platitudes to ease the awkward moments, hoping to avoid exposing our own inadequacies and frailties. During difficult times it may be easier to hide behind our mask of professionalism or busyness than to admit that we do not know all the answers. We cannot solve all the problems and we must have the courage and honesty to tell the patient so.

At times we may have to endure rejection from those we have tried to help. A patient overwhelmed by their illness, their diagnosis, never-ending tests or treatments, may simply want to escape from their pressures and withdraw into themselves for a while.

We need to face our own limitations, and create avenues for renewing our limited resources. It is all too easy to become exhausted from constantly carrying another's burden, from picking up the pieces and trying to make a unified whole out of them. Just as each nurse is equipped to give care to another, so they must remember to give this same loving, uplifting care to themselves in whatever way specifically benefits them. For when nurses are physically, emotionally and spiritually nurtured they are unquestionably able to care for dying patients in a way which will be mutually rewarding, leading to spiritual growth and healing for both the carer and the cared-for.

As nurses, we are liberated and our load becomes lighter when we acknowledge that spiritual needs are at the very heart of our humanity, that to deny them will not only cause spiritual distress, but may exacerbate physical and emotional problems, such as pain or fear. We cannot justify our lack of involvement; by doing so we risk denying our patients their passage to wholeness and healing. This healing is not synonymous with the absence of disease, but rather the state in which the patient comes to a realistic acceptance of their illness and its outcome, is at peace with themselves and significant others, their god and the world around them. They are living in control of their lives and with hope in their hearts, freed from the anger and the bitterness. The quality of their life has improved despite the presence of a physical illness.

We all know how a wound must heal from its base upwards, and not superficially across the top, leaving an empty cavern inside. Similarly, a person, especially one approaching death, may need that deep healing. Physical and emotional care, 'the bread' we give to our patients, may appear to solve all the obvious problems, but unless we probe deeper and reach the heart of the matter, the spiritual side of the person, we leave them with a great unhealed hollow, an emptiness. As nurses it is our duty to help to fill this void, to respond to the spiritual needs of our patients. As they pour out their heart to us, and we respond with compassion, acceptance, honesty and love, walking with them as a friend on their journey, we too are enriched. By drawing closer to them, in some mysterious way we are brought to a new understanding of truth, love, and spirituality; we too, are healed.

REFERENCES

Covey SR (1989): *The Seven Habits of Highly Effective People.* New York: Simon & Schuster.

Doyle D (1983): *Coping with a Dying Relative.* Edinburgh: MacDonald Printers Ltd.

Kübler-Ross E (1970): *On Death and Dying.* London: Tavistock Publications.

Rogers CR (1961): *On Becoming a Person.* Boston: Houghton Mifflin Company.

OTHER READING

Bellemare D and Smyth P (1988): Spirituality, pastoral care and religion: the need for clear distinctions. *Journal of Palliative Care* 4 1-2: 86-88.

Balfour Mount MD (1993): Whole person care: beyond psychosocial and physical needs. *American Journal of Hospice and Palliative Care* January: 28-36.

Campbell AV (1981): *Rediscovering Pastoral Care.* London: Darton Longman & Todd.

Cassidy S (1988): *Sharing the Darkness.* London: Darton Longman & Todd.

Doyle D (1992): Have we looked beyond the physical and psychosocial? *Journal of Pain and Symptom Management* 7 5 July: 302-311.

Drinkwater DJ (ed.) (1974): *Know Thyself.* Sydney: John Wiley & Sons Australasia Pty Ltd.

Eaton S (1988): Spiritual care: the software of life. *Journal of Palliative Care* 4 1-2: 91-93.

Gyulay JE and Karnes B (1984): Healing the dying person. *American Journal of Hospice Care* Fall: 28-32.

Hodder P and Turby A (eds) (1989): *The Creative Option of Palliative Care.* Melbourne: Melbourne Citymission.

Owen-Still S (1985): Spiritual caregiving. *American Journal of Hospice Care* March–April: 32-35.

Schuetz B (1995): Spirituality and palliative care. *Australian Family Physician* May: 775-777.

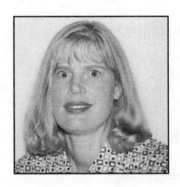

BRIGITTE VAN HEERE
BN (HONOURS), BSc, RN

This chapter is a reflection of the research that Brigitte van Heere undertook as part of the Bachelor of Nursing (Honours) program, under the supervision of Anne Fry, Senior Lecturer in Mental Health Nursing at the University of Western Sydney — Nepean. The research was started after Brigitte finished her Bachelor of Nursing.

Brigitte found that the course constantly reiterated the need to provide holistic nursing care, but there seemed to be a lack of information on how to deal with the spiritual needs of a patient. This lead to the development of such questions in her mind as: 'How am I supposed to care for the spiritual needs of my patients?' and 'How do other nurses look after their patients' spiritual needs?' With these questions running through her mind, she began to look into how nurses attended to their patients' spiritual needs. While conducting this research she worked full time as a registered nurse. At present she is working full time in the Intensive Care/Coronary Care Unit at Campbelltown Hospital in New South Wales.

Chapter 9

SPIRITUAL CARE OF PALLIATIVE CARE PATIENTS

The nursing profession has stated repeatedly that its approach to care is holistic, implying that nursing considers all aspects of a person. That is, nursing cares for the patient's physical, psychosocial and spiritual needs (Taylor, Lillis and LeMone, 1989). However, there are problems with delivering this holistic nursing care, a major problem being that there appears to be little literature available to guide nurses on how to attend to their patients' spiritual needs. This chapter aims to help overcome this problem in two ways: first, by briefly identifying the four spiritual needs, because an understanding of the spiritual needs is important if nurses are to attempt to address these needs; and, secondly, by presenting examples of how spiritual care is delivered by Registered Nurses (RNs) to their palliative care patients. It is hoped that through their examples and by clarification of the skills that are involved more RNs will begin to address their patients' spiritual needs. The skills and spiritual needs addressed in these examples are not unique to palliative care patients; they can be applied to all categories of patients as all patients can experience, albeit from a differing perspective, one or more of the four spiritual needs whilst requiring the assistance of the nursing profession.

SPIRITUAL NEEDS

The theoretical and empirical literature both identify four spiritual needs. These are the search for meaning, a sense of forgiveness, the need for love, and a need for hope (Conrad, 1985; Fish and Shelly, 1978; Highfield and Cason, 1983; Peterson and Nelson, 1987; Schoenbeck, 1994). Any health crisis can trigger spiritual distress and so these needs are not unique to the palliative care patient. Consequently, nurses delivering patient care must be able both to recognise their patients' spiritual needs and to have an understanding of those spiritual needs.

Search for meaning

The search for meaning takes place in us all. As Burnard writes, ' . . . it would appear that most of us need to make sense of our lives in terms of some sort of meaning, but while some invest that meaning through a religious framework, others do not' (1988:130). Thus, as nurses, we need to consider that our own philosophy/meaning of life may not be a universal belief. It is therefore vital that nurses respect the beliefs of their patients. Some patients may have adopted the stance of being atheist or agnostic. Yet, despite their beliefs, both positions provide meaning to people's lives (Burnard, 1988). Consequently, Burnard (1988) exhorts nurses to clarify their own beliefs before they can help their patients. This, combined with an open mind, is vital in helping patients with their search for meaning.

Sense of forgiveness

The next spiritual need is a sense of forgiveness. The patient, in finding meaning in his/her life, may encounter episodes of guilt

(Conrad, 1985; Schoenbeck, 1994). Guilt may be manifested in several ways including anger or the inability to tolerate criticism (Peterson and Nelson, 1987). The reason for this is that some patients are still ruminating over past difficulties, either with people or with certain situations (Conrad, 1985). The nurse needs to recognise the person's guilt and help them to overcome the guilty feeling (Conrad, 1985). As Conrad (1985) notes, people from all belief systems must resolve feelings of guilt towards other human beings and/or in their relationship with another realm.

Need for love

The third spiritual need is the need for love. The source of love will be very personal. Patients can receive love from any human relationships such as friends, family and staff. They can also receive love from their relationship with another realm and this love is very personalised (Conrad, 1985). The need for love must be satisfied; irrespective of how demanding the terminally ill patient may be, they must be given unconditional love (Conrad, 1985; Schoenbeck, 1994).

Hope

Hope is a term that eludes a simplistic definition and no universal definition exists (Herth, 1990; Owen, 1989). Stotland defined hope as 'an expectation of goal attainment modified by the importance of the goal and the probability of attaining it' (cited in Raleigh, 1992:443). It follows that 'the greater the expectation of attaining a goal, the more likely the individual will act in order to attain it' (Stotland, cited in Raleigh, 1992:443). It may seem difficult to instil hope in a terminally ill patient. However, patients can still hope to be in control of their symptoms and treatment. Terminally ill patients can also have an abstract form of hope which deals with life after death (Schoenbeck, 1994). So, as nurses, we cannot necessarily give hope to our patients, but we can encourage it (Simsen, 1988).

PROVIDING SPIRITUAL CARE

Attending to the spiritual needs of the palliative care patient is an important part of providing holistic nursing care, as the palliative care patient has a heightened spiritual awareness. However, there is a dearth of empirical literature available to help guide nurses in delivering spiritual care to their palliative care patients. A descriptive design was utilised to investigate how RNs assess and provide for their patients' spiritual needs. A random sample of 300 RNs were sent a questionnaire which was completed and returned by 75 RNs. Part of the discussion of the research will be presented to both describe and illustrate how RNs provide spiritual care to their patients. The discussion follows the framework of the nursing process.

Assessing and diagnosing

The first step in the nursing process involves the nurse conducting an assessment and diagnosing the patient's problems. It is an important step, as it helps in formulating appropriate nursing care. In assessing the spiritual domain, the RNs used various methods, most commonly through some form of discussion (oral communication) with the patient (listening, the initial interview, and asking the patient about their religion/concerns/spiritual needs) and by observing an exacerbation of either physical or psychological symptoms.

Discussion (oral communication) and observation are the ways with which the RNs assessed and subsequently diagnosed their patients' spiritual distress. While these terms describe what the nurses are doing, they do not illuminate meaning or show how the RNs performed their patient assessment. Nevertheless, examples from the accounts given by the RNs will be used both to illustrate meaning and to describe how these nurses assess and diagnose their patients' spiritual needs through discussion and observation.

Discussion is a term frequently used by the RNs; however, a more accurate description of what the RNs are doing is what Egan (1994) describes as complete listening. Egan (1994) describes complete listening as having four components. 'First, observing and reading the client's nonverbal behaviour . . . Secondly, listening to and understanding the client's verbal messages. Thirdly, listening to the context . . . fourthly, listening to sour notes' (Egan, 1994:94). Complete listening is a difficult skill (Labun, 1988; Burnard, 1990). Nevertheless, complete listening will allow the patient to verbalise concerns (Labun, 1988; Burnard, 1990). Several of the RNs demonstrated that they used some or all of the components of complete listening. In the first example the RN describes what is happening to Mrs S.

Mrs S. had had a long battle with cervical cancer and multiple mets [metastases]. *She has some unusual complications with an intracranial bleed which had caused partial paralysis of her face and arm. She had now developed a large DVT* [deep vein thrombosis] *in the proximal portion of her leg. She had been warned that this clot could fragment at any time and she could have a PE* [pulmonary embolism] *and die immediately. She was beside herself with fear, crying and distraught. I listened to her fears:*

- uncertainty — will the next breath be my last?
- terror of the unknown — what will my death be like?
- loneliness
- bewilderment — why is all this happening?

I discovered that Mrs S. had been a practising Anglican until her husband had died when she abandoned her beliefs because God did not listen to her. However, she had an appropriate framework for me to paint some detail in. We talked . . .

In describing the account of Mrs S., the nurse clearly used all of the components of complete listening. The nurse:

- observed nonverbal behaviours — 'beside herself with fear'
- listened and understood the client's message
- placed the account in context.

The last component of complete listening described by Egan (1994), sour notes, was also noted in the account of Mrs S. — 'I discovered that Mrs S. had been a practising Anglican until her husband had died when she abandoned her beliefs because God did not listen to her'. This challenged the nurse to find out why the patient felt this way. The account given by the RN showed that, through differing cues, the RN identified that the patient had spiritual needs.

The next example also shows an RN using the skill of complete listening to help a patient:

A young man was in turmoil/distress through family estrangements and his lifestyle behaviours. This caused him to be very angry, tearful and in pain that was unable to be managed. I communicated, with him by my patience and willingness to sit and listen to him, an acceptance of his turmoil.

He communicated his distress, his beliefs etc. and through my
acceptance was able to clarify why he was so distressed.

In reviewing the account given by the RN, it is noted that the
RN was again listening to the patient. The RN observed
nonverbal communication by noting that the patient was 'very
angry, tearful'. The second component, listening and
understanding, was also used — 'He communicated his
distress . . .' The RN also put the account in context by
describing the scenario: 'A young man was in turmoil/distress
through family estrangements and his lifestyle behaviours'.
The RN also identified the sour notes in the young man's story.
In addition the RN illustrated other qualities which helped
develop the nurse–patient relationship, qualities such as having
both a nonjudgemental attitude and accepting the patient's
turmoil which resulted from the patient's lifestyle. These
qualities are important if they mean that the patient will fully
disclose herself/himself to the nurse.

Another communication skill employed by one of the RNs
was that of helping the patient to tell their life story:

A 72 year old man with cancer who found it difficult to
understand how he, who had never done anyone any harm,
worked hard, loved his family, never smoked or drank, could get
cancer and now have to leave his wife who didn't deserve to be
left alone. I asked him to tell me his life story interjecting happily
on all the joyous and positive aspects. He relaxed and we had
some laughs and tears and at the closing he once again looked
puzzled, asking 'Why? Why?'

In telling his life story, the patient told the nurse the
problems he had. This allowed the nurse to view the problems
in context, observe nonverbal cues, listen to the oral message

and take note of what might need to be challenged. In so doing a relationship between the patient and nurse was developed.

The next method employed by the RNs for assessing a patient's spiritual needs was by observing an exacerbation of symptoms. It is debatable if an exacerbation of physical and/or psychological symptoms is a way of discerning spiritual needs. Nevertheless, the RNs indicated that this was a method of assessing a patient for spiritual needs, an idea that could find support when viewing the person from a holistic perspective. That is, 'our beings, body, mind, and spiritual, are dynamically woven together, one part affecting and being affected by the other parts' (Stoll, 1989:8). This idea is reinforced by Reed's comments that 'Components of spirituality cross traditional science boundaries such that the spiritual cannot be distinguished necessarily from what has been labelled as social, psychological or physical parts of a human being' (Reed, 1992:354-355). Labun's definition of spirituality also lends support for the idea that an exacerbation of physical and psychological symptoms could be a result of the patient experiencing spiritual distress. Labun states that spirituality is 'an aspect of the total person which is related to and integrated with the functioning and expression of all other aspects of the person' (1988:315). It follows that spiritual distress is a 'disruption in the life principle that pervades a person's entire being and that integrates and transcends one's biological and psychosocial nature' (Kim et al., cited in Labun, 1988:318), supporting the premise that spiritual distress can be diagnosed from observing an exacerbation of either physical or psychological symptoms.

Debating whether an exacerbation of symptoms such as pain or anxiety can indicate spiritual distress is beyond the scope of this chapter. Nevertheless, there is support for the idea. The RNs indicated that, by observing an exacerbation of symptoms, they are able to diagnose spiritual distress. However, this alone does not provide meaning. To instil meaning, some accounts will be given to further illustrate how the nurse identifies spiritual distress from an exacerbation of symptoms. The first account:

A 55 year old man was admitted for care in his last week or two. In obvious distress from unrelieved pain. When pain relief administered and patient still not 100% pain free I asked him if there were any problems (other than physical ones) that were worrying him. He told me that he was really concerned that he had not practised his religion (Roman Catholic) for many years and was worried that he may be sent to purgatory. Not being a RC [Roman Catholic] myself and having no real understanding of the religion I asked a member of the pastoral care team who was a nun to speak with the man. After this, the man seemed far more relaxed and his pain levels went down also so that the narcotic drug could be reduced.

The nurse observed that the pain was not just physical pain, but spiritual. After attending to the patient's spiritual needs the symptom (pain) decreased.

The second example again illustrates the necessity of providing spiritual care to help alleviate other symptoms:

Michael was a young man with osteosarcoma who, following a horrendous time in a hospital, returned to our regional hospital a paraplegic and facing death. Pain was his main problem but absolutely nothing worked and it became obvious that his pain was spiritual. None of us could break through the barrier so we arranged — with Michael's permission, of course — to get a

Buddhist monk to visit. This happened and Michael immediately gained some pain relief with peace of mind.

Again, after spiritual care was given, the patient had a decrease in symptoms and attained peace of mind.

A decrease in symptoms happened not only to Michael but also in the following account:

> *. . . a Catholic who was married to a doctor. She converted to Anglican before marriage . . . the patient, dying, asked for a Catholic priest. The patient was very agitated and in a lot of pain. Priest visited three times or so and the woman converted back to Catholicism. She became peaceful, pain better controlled.*

These three examples all show that the RNs identified spiritual distress by observing an exacerbation of physical and/or psychological symptoms. When provided with spiritual care the patients attained a sense of peace and their symptoms were minimised. Therefore, it could be concluded that the provision of spiritual care can lead to the attainment of peace and a subsequent decrease in the severity of symptoms.

Planning and implementation

Having identified the patient's spiritual needs, the next important step in the nursing process is that of planning and implementing strategies to eliminate the spiritual need(s). Having identified that the patient has a spiritual need or needs it is assumed that the goal would be to fulfil the spiritual need(s) or eliminate the spiritual distress.

In providing spiritual care to their patients, the majority (62.7 per cent) of RNs stated that they refer their patients either to pastoral care or to the clergy, instead of dealing with the spiritual issues themselves. It could be speculated that the reason behind the majority of the RNs referring their patients either to pastoral care or to the clergy is that perhaps nurses have insufficient time to deal with their patients' spiritual issues. However, these resource people are not always available after hours when many of these problems surface. So exclusive dependence on either the clergy or pastoral care to provide continuous spiritual care is not always feasible. Therefore a 'caring environment should be in place to enhance and promote spiritual work at any time, not just at designated times'(Corless et al., 1990:77).

Although the majority of RNs refer their patients to either pastoral care or to the clergy, several RNs gave narratives illustrating how they had provided spiritual care to a patient in the past. The following two accounts illustrate how two RNs gave spiritual care to their respective patients:

A 49 year old bowel cancer lady who lost her husband 8 months earlier with a haemorrhage . . . is very frightened about her impending death . . . She is very depressed. I visited her one day . . . she started to cry and showed me a poster on her bedroom wall of a beautiful waterfall. This was the place that her and her husband said they would meet when they both died. When she bought the poster it had no marks on it but now it has 2 marks near the water's edge that are similar to people. She informed me that these marks are getting darker and she believes it is a sign her husband is waiting for her. I encouraged this belief and talked about experiences I've had with other dying people who talk to loved ones or see loved ones before they die. This was important to this lady because it gave her a sense of peace and something to hold onto as she gets closer to death.

A 38 year old male, who I will call Mark, had cancer of the pancreas. He was very agitated one day. His pain had been well controlled but suddenly escalated. He was very restless and after a breakthrough dose of Morphine he started talking about how he wanted to be at peace with himself. He stated he had been raised as a Catholic, but had not practised for years. He then went on to explain his theories and how he had always wanted to meditate, but did not know how. Mark asked me if I'd ever meditated and I told him about an Ashram I used to attend in the 80s, where I took meditation 'lessons'. We discussed basic principles and I was able to loan Mark some of the ward's tapes. He asked if there was a local person who would visit the hospital to give him lessons. Through a local network Mark was able to choose a teacher. She visited him regularly for lessons and Mark, over time, achieved peace with himself.

The two RNs clearly used many of the communication skills mentioned previously to either instil hope or help the patient overcome feelings of guilt. The RNs also clearly used self-disclosure to help their patients, for example, '. . . talked about experiences I've had with other dying people' and 'I told him about an Ashram I used to attend . . . ' According to Amenta: 'In effective spiritual support judicious use of self-disclosure is appropriate. Worker and afflicted person become partners in dialogue' (1988:51). These two examples illustrate the RNs' use of self-disclosure.

Through delivering spiritual care, other RNs showed the depth of the nurse–patient relationship. The following examples show the depth of the caring relationship that can develop as nurses go beyond what is considered their role/duty:

Mrs M., who was a regular church attendant, was unable to read the passage in her bible each day. I would read this to her in my morning tea break and we often talked about it afterwards and what it offered her in particular. The minister was often phoned by staff at Mrs M.'s request and family were kept informed of her progress. Both her will and funeral arrangements were discussed with family but she often shared these personal choices with me for reassurance. We prayed together often.

A patient that had no religion in his life wanted to be baptised and convert to Catholicism before he died. His wife had no formal religion but backed his wishes. I organised transport there and back, went on my day off and showered and dressed him to make it easier on all. He seemed at peace afterwards and went very quickly and almost painfree.

A 41 year old man, a father of 6, estranged from wife — she kept the kids and 'ran off' with his best mate — I helped him to explore his feelings/questions, to 'whip' anger . . . Many many 'deep and meaningful' chats with him (by me) and all our staff . . . Basically sat and listened to Mark and his thoughts (anger re: pain and dying), 'I'm not ready'. Myself and wardsman, after Mark's death, did not put him into the [mortuary] fridge but gave his body to the funeral director, to their van, and they promised they'd put him in their 'cool room' not into a small fridge. Mark was claustrophobic. So Henry and I kept our last promise to Mark.

One other patient who I learnt from was 26 with a young family. I had only been in palliative care a few weeks when one night he asked me how long he had till he died. I was dumbfounded but asked him how long he thought he had.

He told me he would be dead by Tuesday (a few days away).
He talked about his son (6 months old) and that he wanted to
leave him something as he was completing a colouring-in book
and he would be finished it by Tuesday. We talked for a while,
he asked me that if his young wife couldn't sit with him when
he was dying, could I promise him I would stay with him. I
promised him this. A few days later he deteriorated so I went
to the unit (as I was on days off). I went and spoke with his
family and sat with them and Robert for more than an hour. I
then said goodbye to Robert (he was now unconscious) and
told him the promise was that I would be there if his wife
couldn't stay but she wanted to stay with him and so I wasn't
needed. I then left. Robert died peacefully within the hour. He
would tell me he visualised himself surfing all his life — he even
had us filling up the spa bath with cold water when he had been
well enough.

The stories of these four RNs illustrate how they developed
a very caring relationship with their patients which was
beyond the call of duty. One RN spent tea breaks with the
patient to read the Bible. Another RN came in on days off to
allow the patient to convert back to Catholicism. The last
two RNs showed their integrity by keeping the promises that
they had made to their respective patients. Their actions all
facilitated their patients in overcoming spiritual distress, so
enabling them to attain peace and alleviate fears.

Evaluation

The final step in the nursing process is evaluation. In
evaluating nursing care it is hoped that the nurse will either
find that the care is complete, or revise some of the strategies
to eliminate the spiritual needs faced by the patient. The RNs
who returned their questionnaires, in evaluating their

delivery of spiritual care, noted that they asked their patients if their needs had been met. Another indicator employed to measure the effectiveness of spiritual care, was by observing their patients' peaceful appearance and/or death. The RNs noted that peace was an outcome that was attained after spiritual care had been provided. A summary of some of the ways in which the term 'peace' was used by the RNs runs as follows:

Once the priest left he fell into a peaceful state of unconsciousness . . . The wife states she was sure he was at peace.

Peaceful, he faced his maker in death.

The man did not suffer any pain and was completely relaxed and 'peaceful' when he died 3 days later.

. . . slept peacefully that night and died the next day.

He died at peace, feeling forgiven.

A peace came over the daughter and she fell asleep — her pain and suffering over. The mother thanked me for my compassion and understanding.

He then died a peaceful death.

Robert died peacefully within the hour.

At least they went peacefully.

Although the aim may be to attain peace at death, the question that needs to be asked is, what happens if the death is not peaceful? Could the death have been peaceful if the strategies had been evaluated earlier? Or is peace the goal of the nursing strategies in eliminating spiritual distress? Lederer et al. (1991) do not mention the concept of peace as an outcome of relief of spiritual distress. Still, the RNs rank it as an important way of measuring that their patients' spiritual distress had been alleviated/minimised. Nevertheless, evaluating the effectiveness of nursing care by observing how the patient died would appear to be a bit late if the strategies needed re-evaluating.

Some of the RNs stated that they either did not evaluate the spiritual care given or did so with great difficulty. This could be a reflection that the entire concept of spirituality is a difficult topic for nurses to deal with. Maybe nurses have problems with their own spirituality. 'Nurses need first to clarify their own beliefs and value systems before they can help patients with such ultimate questions' (Burnard, 1988:132). In other words, 'Know thyself' (Conrad, 1985:419).

CONCLUSION

Attending to the patient's spiritual needs involves the use of some complex communication skills. However, it is perhaps more important to remember that not everyone shares the same view on spirituality. In providing spiritual care nurses should have a broad understanding of spirituality. This understanding will enable the nurse to deal with patients' ultimate questions (Burnard, 1987; Conrad, 1985). Also, in having a nonjudgemental and open mind, the nurse will be in a better position to help the patient. Burnard (1987) also advocates that, before helping a patient, it is important for the nurse to sort out her or his own views on life so as not to feel threatened by the views of others. This will make the nurse more effective in being a provider of spiritual care. In other words, 'Know thyself' (Conrad, 1985:419). Once this is established, and the nurse has an understanding of what spiritual needs are, it is envisaged that, with increased experience, RNs will gain confidence in attending to their patients' spiritual needs.

REFERENCES

Amenta M (1988): Nurses as primary spiritual care workers. *Hospice Journal* 4: 47-55.

Burnard P (1987): Spiritual distress and the nursing response: Theoretical consider-ations and counselling skills. *Journal of Advanced Nursing* 12: 377-382.

Burnard P (1988): The spiritual needs of atheists and agnostics. *Professional Nurse* 4: 130-132.

Burnard P (1990): Learning to care for the spirit. *Nursing Standard* 4: 38-39.

Conrad N (1985): Spiritual support for the dying. *Nursing Clinics of North America* 20: 415-426.

Corless I, Wald F, Autton CN, Bailey S, Cosh R, Cockburn M, Head D, DeVeber B, DeVeber I, Ley DCH, Mauritzen J, Nichols J, O'Connor P, Saito T (1990): Assumptions and principles of spiritual care. *Death Studies* 14: 75-81.

Egan G (1994): *The Skilled Helper: A Problem Management Approach to Helping* (5th edn). Pacific Grove, California: Brooks/Cole Publishing Company.

Fish S and Shelly JA (1978): *Spiritual Care: Nurse's Role.* Downers Grove, Illinois: Intervarsity Press.

Herth KA (1990): Fostering hope in terminally-ill people. *Journal of Advanced Nursing* 15: 1250-1259.

Highfield MF and Cason C (1983): Spiritual needs of patients: Are they recognised? *Cancer Nursing* 6: 187-92.

Labun E (1988): Spiritual care: an element in nursing care planning. *Journal of Advanced Nursing* 13: 314-320.

Lederer JR, Marculescu GL, Mocnik B, Seaby N (1991): *Care Planning Pocket Guide. A Nursing Approach* (4th edn). Redwood City, California: Addison-Wesley Nursing.

Owen DC (1989): Nurses' perspectives on the meaning of hope in patients with cancer: A qualitative study. *Oncology Nursing Forum* 16: 75-79.

Peterson EA and Nelson K (1987): How to meet your client's spiritual needs. *Journal of Psychosocial Nursing* 25: 34-39.

Raleigh EDH (1992): Sources of hope in chronic illness. *Oncology Nursing Forum* 19: 443-448.

Reed PG (1992): An emerging paradigm for the investigation of spirituality in nursing. *Research in Nursing and Health* 15: 349-357.

Schoenbeck SL (1994): Called to care: Addressing the spiritual needs of patients. *Journal of Practical Nursing* 44: 19-23.

Simsen B (1988): Nursing the spirit. *Nursing Times* 84: 32-33.

Stoll R (1989): The essence of spirituality. In: Carson VB (ed.): *Spiritual Dimensions of Nursing Practice*. Philadelphia: WB Saunders, pp. 4-23.

Taylor C, Lillis C, LeMone P (1989): *Fundamentals of Nursing Care: The Art and Science of Nursing*. Philadelphia: JB Lippincott Company.

INDEX